D0893248

COUNTRY DOCTOR

AND

CITY DOCTOR
FATHER AND DAUGHTER

Theresa Brey Haddy, M.D.

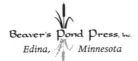
Beaver's Pond Press, Inc.
Edina, Minnesota

ISBN 13: 978-1-59298-151-9
ISBN 10: 1-59298-151-8

Library of Congress Catalog Number: 2006926132

Book design and typesetting: Mori Studio, Inc.
Cover design: Mori Studio, Inc.

Printed in the United States of America

First Printing: April 2006

10 09 08 07 06   5 4 3 2 1

Beaver's Pond Press, Inc.   7104 Ohms Lane, Suite 216
Edina, MN 55439
(952) 829-8818
www.BeaversPondPress.com

To order, visit www.BookHouseFulfillment.com or call
1-800-901-3480. Reseller and special sales discounts available.

This Book is Dedicated

To Fran, who never met his father-in-law;
Rick, Carol, and Alice,
who never knew their maternal grandfather;
and
Ann, who helped make it possible.

CONTENTS

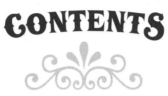

ACKNOWLEDGEMENTS

I owe a great deal to my sister, Ann Catherine Brey, who maintained my father's records, photographs, and belongings over many years, so that they were available when I came to write this book. Thanks are due also to my son, Richard Ian Haddy, M.D., who analyzed data from Dr. Frank W. Brey's daybooks and compared my father's family practice in Minnesota during the early twentieth century to his own contemporary family practice in Ohio. Jodi Johnston's biography of my husband's father, Thomas Joseph Haddy (Patriarch: The Life of T. J. Haddy, Noble House, Baltimore, 1994), inspired me to write about my own father. Jacalyn Duffin's book about a physician who practiced medicine in Canada during the late nineteenth century (Langstaff: A Nineteenth-Century Medical Life, University of Toronto Press, Toronto, 1993) was an additional source of inspiration to me.

Those who remembered my father or reminisced about earlier times were, first and foremost, my sisters and brothers, Ann Catherine Brey, Alois John Brey, Virginia Brey Osterbauer, Paul Daub Brey, and Justine Brey DuBruil. Other relatives and friends included Ludwig Daub, Robert Daub, Beatrice Fixsen Emmerick, Ambrose J. Schmelzle, Ph.D, Myrtle Schmelzle, Arlean Schwing, and Belva Emmerick Wilkinson.

Among the many other people who helped were Dorothy Boehm, Student Relations, University of Minnesota, Minneapolis, Minnesota; Robert Burgett, Associate Vice President for Development, Minnesota

Medical Foundation, Minneapolis, Minnesota; Paul E. Birk, Jr., M.D., Glenview, Illinois; Patricia R. Conard, M.D., Glenview, Illinois; Gail Finley, Medical Examiners Office, Redwood Falls, Minnesota; James Flinn, M.D., retired Medical Examiner, Redwood Falls, Minnesota; John Hagan, Court Administrator, Redwood County Court, Redwood Falls, Minnesota; Paul Jarosinski, Clinical Pharmacy Specialist and Coordinator, National Institutes of Health, Bethesda, Maryland; Jude Johnson, librarian, Redwood Falls, Minnesota; Scott D. McGinnis, research consultant, Donivan Research, Plymouth, Minnesota; personnel at the Minnesota Historical Society; Morris Osterbauer, pharmacist (and brother-in-law), Rice Lake, Wisconsin; Patrick E. Shields, Ph.D., Director of Development, Department of Pediatrics, University of Minnesota, Minneapolis, Minnesota; and Robert D. Tiegs, M.D., Mayo Clinic, Rochester, Minnesota.

INTRODUCTION

My father, Frank W. Brey, M.D., was an old-time family physician who had a solo family practice in a small town in southern Minnesota from 1910 to 1940. He was a respected member of his profession, a leader in the community, a devoted husband and father, and the most important influence in my early years. The original title of my book was "He Always Came" because he always came when a patient called him. If the weather was severe, even in the midst of a blinding snowstorm or a blizzard, he always came. If it was in the middle of the night or on the weekend, he always came. If the patient was unable or unwilling to pay, he always came. After I decided to include something of myself in the book, the original title was no longer appropriate, and was changed to "Country Doctor and City Doctor: Father and Daughter" in order to include me and indicate the disparity of time between us and the places where we worked.

I was young when my father died—sixteen years old—but my memory of him is clear. This memoir is reconstructed from my own memory, as well as from interviews with family and friends, documents he left behind, and various published materials. My sister Ann has preserved his papers, photographs, books, duck decoys, a buffalo coat, and even a tapeworm, tucked away in the attic of my family home.

FRONTIER MEDICINE

My father was typical of his time, and his story, which concerns frontier medicine in the first part of the twentieth century, was similar to those of many other early rural physicians. They were pioneers in the practice of medicine who had to rely upon their own abilities, their ingenuity, and above all, their courage. They worked without diagnostic x-rays and laboratory tests, lacked modern pharmaceutical agents, often had no close colleague with whom to exchange advice and emergency calls, and sometimes faced adverse weather conditions while making house calls. As physicians, they were concerned about how to keep up with new medical developments. Most of all, the serious diseases and injuries that they periodically encountered but were not equipped to manage satisfactorily must have been an ongoing source of distress.

In dealing with day to day medical and surgical problems, emergencies, and life-threatening situations, my father was on his own without nursing assistance at first, with no available pharmacist in the early years, and without a nearby hospital or emergency room. There was no close colleague with whom to consult and discuss problems. He was constantly on call, with no days off and no vacations. The local physician was expected to do his duty and be available; there was no talk of "burn-out" in those days. Often nothing could be done for a patient except to "be there." Because he always came when he was called, my father was respected and appreciated by the community. He was strong and dependable, devoted to his family, and compassionate toward the poor and the sick.

My father's story covers the fifty-four years of his life and his thirty years as a country doctor in Wabasso, Minnesota, until his death in the spring of 1940. He lived during the last fourteen years of the nineteenth century and the first four decades of the twentieth century, but his story starts before that, with the Great Plains of southern Minnesota and the pioneers who settled there. He died at a time when physicians were no longer being attracted to rural practices and villages, and small towns were being left without easily available medical care. My father's practice was taken over for a few years by several other physicians who came and went, but Wabasso, like many other small towns, does not now have a physician who lives and practices there.

BIG CITY MEDICINE

I have been a pediatric hematologist/oncologist, centered on the treatment of children with diseases of the blood and cancer, throughout most of my medical career. Much of my medical training and practice was in large city hospitals in Minneapolis, Oklahoma City, and the District of Columbia, but some of my experience has been in small towns, too. I was a partner in a general pediatric practice in the Chicago suburbs of Arlington Heights and Des Plaines, and my pediatric hematology/oncology practice in Michigan was in the Lansing community hospitals. Because children with diseases of the blood and cancer need to be hospitalized frequently, a pediatric hematologist/oncologist functions to a large extent using hospital care.

My own story starts in 1940, the year of my father's death, the year when I turned sixteen and went away to school to learn to be a doctor. Very few women studied medicine in those days, and I had met only one woman physician, so I had no idea about what to expect. At first I had to deal with a good deal of discrimination against women entering the medical field, but this attitude became less throughout the years. Women are not only well accepted these days, but there are equal numbers of them and sometimes even a majority in medical schools.

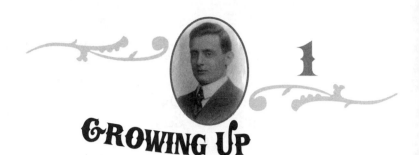

GROWING UP

IN SOUTHERN MINNESOTA
1886-1905

n the early nineteenth century almost nothing was known about infectious diseases, and the "germ theory" had not yet been developed. Parasitic infestations with tapeworm, hookworm, and trichinosis had been identified, but bacteria were not discovered until later. Oliver Wendell Holmes wrote in 1843 that an infectious agent probably caused childbed fever, but his suggestion was not well received. The use of cowpox vaccine to immunize people against smallpox had been introduced into the United States in 1800, but other forms of immunization were not discovered until the end of the century. By the second half of the nineteenth century, bloodletting with a lance, cupping, the use of violent emetics to cause vomiting, and the purging of the bowels by enemas or toxic chemicals were falling into disrepute. Such "heroic therapy" continued to some extent, however, even into the twentieth century. Opiates, containing or derived from opium, were easily available with or without prescription, and alcohol was freely advocated for a wide variety of complaints. Anthrax, tuberculosis, and cholera bacilli were identified. X-rays were discovered by Wilhelm Roentgen in Germany in 1895, and radium was isolated by Pierre and Marie Curie in France in 1898. Working in Vienna, Karl Landsteiner identified blood groups in 1901 and thus laid the foundation for safe blood transfusions and modern blood banking.

My father, Francis William Brey, was born in 1886 and brought up on a farm near Lafayette, in Nicollet County, Minnesota. The farm was not far from New Ulm, and his parents eventually retired to a home in New Ulm. Brown County was established in 1855, and the town of New Ulm was founded in 1857 by the German Land Association of Minnesota on the south bank of the Minnesota River in Brown County, just above the mouth of the Cottonwood River.

THE GREAT PLAINS

When my paternal (and maternal) forebears arrived at the exact center of the continent of North America, they found a vast, treeless, prairie wilderness.[1,2] Minnesota is often thought of as being covered with pine or evergreen trees, but in fact the flat plains of the south contrast markedly with the dense forests of the north. When Minnesota became a territory in 1849, the Great Plains, a wide tallgrass prairie, stretched from border to border in the lower third of the state, and pushed up into Canada along its western edge. There were rivers, lakes, and marshes, the only wooded areas being found near rivers, which served as fire breaks. Prairie fires roared across the plains at fairly regular intervals and destroyed any trees that tried to grow on the prairie. Fires were usually started by lightning but were sometimes set by Native Americans who wanted to flush game or attract game to the new grass growth that quickly followed the burn-off.

The tall grasses that characterized the eastern belt of the Minnesota Great Plains consisted of Indian grass, switchgrass, and big bluestem grasses. The herds of bison that roamed the prairie wilderness were sometimes almost hidden by the tall grasses, which could reach as high as six to 12 feet in years when the rainfall was good. There were also elk, antelope, foxes, wolves, rabbits, deermice, and many other animals. Large numbers of prairie chickens lived among the long, wavy grasses, and hawks and meadowlarks were abundant. The prairie pothole region, which included southwestern Minnesota, offered prime nesting and rearing sites for many ducks. Wild rice grew in marshy wetlands, and the rivers and lakes contained many varieties of fish.

Waterways were the natural means of transportation, and the Minnesota River was the highway west for my ancestors, as it was for many other immigrants. From the western border of the state, the river flowed southeast across lower Minnesota for two-thirds of its length, made a sharp bend to the northeast at Mankato, and emptied into the Mississippi River at Saint Paul. The towns of Mankato, Red Wing, and Wabasha, all named after Sioux chiefs, already existed. Travelers went by boat up the Minnesota River and, in the case of my mother's family, even further up its tributary, the Redwood River, to where they would finally settle on the Great Plains of southwestern Minnesota.

FRONTIER ALONG THE MINNESOTA RIVER

The New Ulm-Redwood Falls area where my grandparents and great grandparents settled remained largely unexplored until 1850, when the steamboat *Yankee* proceeded up the Minnesota River as far as its junction with the Cottonwood River. At that time only a few fur trappers and isolated groups of Native Americans were to be found on the Northern Great Plains, most of them near rivers. The Sioux (Dakota) Indians had previously lived in eastern Minnesota, close to the Mississippi River. They were nomadic hunters and fishers who ate mostly venison and wild rice. The Chippewa (Ojibway) Indians, who were the bitter enemies of the Sioux, lived in forested areas to the north and east.

In 1851 the Sioux signed away their rights to their ancestral hunting grounds, and by 1853 most of the Indians had moved to reservations, Fort Ridgely was built, and the way was open to white settlers. The fort was intended to house and protect the agency administrators. Situated below the Lower Sioux Agency, the fort was built on the north bank of the Minnesota River in the western corner of Nicollet County (the county in which my paternal grandparents would settle).

THE SIOUX UPRISING OF 1862

My relatives settled in the areas where the Sioux Uprising of 1862 had taken place, my mother's family in the Redwood Falls area near where the uprising began and my father's family in the New Ulm area where the uprising ended. The Sioux Indians, led by Chief Little Crow, attacked white settlers along the Minnesota River in August of 1862, and carried out one of the bloodiest massacres of civilians that ever took place in the United States.

NEW ULM

New Ulm, the largest town in the area at that time, had a population of 635 people in 1860, most of them German immigrants. The town quickly became packed with refugees, and in spite of having very little in the way of munitions, it was successfully defended twice by the townspeople. They fought off the first, relatively mild, assault on August 19, the day before the attack on Fort Ridgely. By the time of the much more serious second attack on August 23 and 24, they had strengthened the barricades raised before the first attack, and various units of armed civilian militia had arrived to increase the town's fighting force. Dr. William Warrell Mayo joined a number of physicians from neighboring towns in setting up hospitals for the sick and wounded. On the day after the second attack was repulsed, 2000 refugees in 153 wagons, escorted by troops that had newly arrived, left the overcrowded town and made it safely to Mankato.

A surrender was negotiated on September 26, 1862. Two days later a military tribunal convened at Camp Release to try 303 captured Indians, who were subsequently transferred to a prison stockade in Mankato.

EXECUTION AT MANKATO

After being tried, 303 captured warriors were convicted and sentenced to death. President Abraham Lincoln reviewed the list and commuted the sentences of all but 38 of the prisoners. They were hanged simultaneously in Mankato on December 26, in the largest official mass execution in United States history. Among the thousands of people who came to witness the hangings were a large number of physicians who hoped to acquire bodies for dissection. At that time there was no formal mechanism to provide cadavers for anatomical studies, and physicians had no choice but to find material for examination as best they could. Medical schools needed bodies to teach anatomy, and many schools relied upon "body snatchers" or "resurrectionists" for cadavers. This led to some illegal practices, and sometimes a family felt that it was necessary to hire a watcher at the cemetery for several nights following a funeral in order to prevent grave-robbing. This situation caused resentment against the medical schools and the medical profession, resentment so pronounced that medical school buildings were burned by mobs in Maryland and Virginia. Public outrage led finally to legislation that allowed medical schools to obtain cadavers without going outside the law. Massachusetts was the first state to legalize the granting of bodies to medical schools in 1830, but some states did not pass an anatomy act until the nineteenth century was almost over.

CUT NOSE AND DR. MAYO

Dr. Mayo, then practicing in LeSeuer, and probably the most prominent physician in attendance, was allotted the body of an Indian named Cut Nose, who was said to be one of the most aggressive and vicious of the attackers. His name came from his physical appearance: one of his nostrils had been bitten off during a fight. Ironically, this same Indian, along with two drunken comrades, had encountered Dr. Mayo on a previous occasion, when he was returning from a housecall.[3] The Indians demanded his horse, but Dr. Mayo escaped without giving it up. The body of Cut Nose was taken to LeSeuer and dissected in the presence of several other physicians. Dr. Mayo moved to Rochester in 1864[3], where he and his sons, William James and Charles Horace, established the Mayo Clinic. The bones of Cut Nose were cleaned and articulated, and it was said that young Will and Charlie learned osteology, which is the scientific study of bones, from the skeleton of Cut Nose. The skeleton became well known around the Mayo Clinic, being kept in Dr. Mayo's office at first and later banished to the brace-building shop, where it was used to make measurements.

GENERATIONAL MEMORIES

When I was a child, my father often took the family to visit his parents in New Ulm, where they lived after they retired from the farm. We could see Fort Ridgely across the river as we drove along the south bank of the Minnesota River, and my father always commented upon the fort. I remember being frightened by bison in one of the local parks, even though they were safely behind strong fences, and my sister Virginia remembers watching Fourth of July parades in New Ulm in which Indians participated, wearing war bonnets and full regalia. At that time these experiences had no historical meaning for me.

So it was most interesting for me to visit New Ulm again, in 1996, and look at the town with a fresh viewpoint. I was surprised to learn from my cousin, Arlean Schwing, who lived there, how closely many of the citizens of the town hold the memories of the Sioux Uprising. As she guided my husband and me around New Ulm, we saw several memorials to the settlers who were killed. Four brick sculptures in an alleyway at 16 North Minnesota Street, "The Settlers," show what the life of the early German settlers and the Dakota Indians was like in the 1850s before the Uprising took place, and in the boulevard at Center and State Streets stands "The Defenders" monument, which honors those who died during the siege. A prominent monument in the Catholic cemetery, where my grandparents and other relatives are buried, is dedicated to "The Pioneers" who gave their lives defending New Ulm. She told us that at least one local business with the word Sioux in its title had been boycotted by the townspeople and had failed simply because of the name. When we teased Arlean, who was in her eighties, about being "politically incorrect," she told us that a number of my paternal grandmother's relatives, the branch of the family to which she belonged, were living in the United States before the Civil War. She said, "When one grows up hearing repeatedly, from early childhood, about how loved ones were killed so brutally in the Uprising, it is impossible to avoid having some resentment."

The generational memory of many people in New Ulm, handed down from their forebears, includes the knowledge that among the whites, counting both civilians and the military, the number of dead was at between 400 and 500, some sources say as many as 800. Twenty-one Sioux were reported killed in battles, but the true number will never be known because the Indians customarily removed their dead from battlefields. The fighting was controlled fairly quickly, ending with the Indians' surrender on September 26, 1862. However, it was the start of the Indian Wars, which were not over until the final Battle of Wounded Knee Creek was fought in South Dakota in 1890. Frightened by the loss of life and widespread property damage, many settlers fled to the east. Many Indians who were not involved in the conflict also fled, fearing that they would be blamed and attacked by whites. As a result, the area suffered for decades from devastation and depopulation. The Sioux were banished from Minnesota, but the bitter feelings between whites and Indians lasted for many years. Very likely, my father's father could afford to purchase his farm in 1875 because the land values must surely have plummeted when so many people left.

THE ALTMANN FAMILY

My father's mother, Anna Altmann, was born in Neumarkt, which is located near Nuremberg in western Germany, on July 4, 1859; she came to Renville County as a nine-year-old child with her parents, Joseph and Theresia. They immigrated in 1868, only six years after the Indian uprising and three years after the end of the Civil War. Two years later, at the time of the 1870 United States census, the family appeared to be doing well. Joseph Altmann was credited with owning a farm near Lafayette worth $2,200, of which 40 acres were improved, that is, under cultivation, and 120 acres were unimproved. Five acres were wetlands; these were probably counted as part of the 120 unimproved acres, since many farms at that time consisted of a quarter section (160 acres) of land, the usual size of a land claim made by a homesteader. Joseph probably purchased, rather than homesteaded, his farm. He owned 52 swine, six cattle (of which two were milk cows), and two horses, with a total value of $310 for all livestock. He also owned farming implements and machinery worth $30, and he had paid out in wages, including board, $15. The farm had produced 12 bushels of spring wheat, 30 of Indian corn, 150 of oats, and 100 of barley, with a total farm production for the year of $935. Five years later, the 1875 census listed Anna living at home as a 16-year-old girl with her father, age 56; mother, age 52; brothers John, age 26, and Franz, age 21; and sisters Maria, age 24, and Theresa, age nine.

The Brey Family

My father's father, Alouis (Alois) Brey, was born in Neumarkt, western Germany, on March 22, 1858. He was one of the three sons born to Joseph Brey and his first wife, Theresia. Joseph's second wife died at a young age, presumably without having children, and he and his third wife had two children, Joseph and Barbara. Alois arrived in the United States in 1875 at 17 years of age, having immigrated with his brothers, Wenzel, who accompanied him to Minnesota, and Anton, who remained in Wisconsin near the site of their immigration. According to my cousin Ambrose (Andy) Schmelzle, whose grandfather was Anton Brey, the three brothers traveled down the St. Lawrence Seaway with three friends, landing in northeastern Wisconsin after a boat trip through the Great Lakes. The last name of one of the friends was Altmann; it is not known whether he was related to the Anna Altmann whom my grandfather later married. Of the other two friends, the last name of one was probably Zettel and the other's was possibly Bretl. Andy's impression was, "They wanted to come to this country to seek their fortunes, yes, but they also wanted to avoid military service in the Austro-Hungarian army."

A good many of the German-speaking people in the area had arrived by boat and disembarked on the shore of Lake Michigan. Andy said, "One of the landing ports was Algoma, Wisconsin, which at that time, I believe, was a village called Ahnapee. There is some indication that my grandfather actually disembarked at Mimtown, about 50 miles south of Algoma. It is likely that he made his way to Algoma and went from there by barge on the Wolf River to the village of Forestville, about six miles west of Algoma. My grandfather, Anton, and two of the friends liked it there and wanted to stay. The Anton Brey homestead is about three miles west of Forestville, between Forestville and Maplewood, and about 12 miles southwest of Sturgeon Bay, Wisconsin. Anton's two brothers and the other friend, whose last name was Altmann, had heard of prairie land that didn't need to be cleared being available in Minnesota, so they went on to southwestern Minnesota to settle around the New Ulm area."

Andy described a touching episode that concerned my grandfather Alois Brey's much younger half-brother, Joseph Brey, who came to the United States at a later date. The deceit he encountered after his arrival here, when a customs agent bought him a railroad ticket that took him only part of the way to his destination, no doubt pocketing the remainder of the money, was not an unusual experience for a new immigrant. The kind assistance he received from strangers was probably not unusual, either.

"This is the story that he related to me," said Andy. "Joe had always hoped to come to America because he had known about his half-brothers being here. When he was twelve years old, the brothers in southwestern Minnesota sent him money so that he could come to this country. He vividly remembered walking to the railroad station with his mother. He had his tickets in his pocket and his mother had given him five dollars, which she sewed into his jacket so that he would have a little extra money. First he traveled by train, and then he got on a boat, I believe in Holland. He sailed across the ocean and eventually arrived in New York.

"The customs agent in New York looked at his papers and said, 'You want to go to Minnesota?'

"The boy couldn't speak English, so there must have been an interpreter present. He answered, 'Ya.'

"'That's fine,' said the agent, 'but it'll cost you five dollars.'

"That didn't worry Joe. He had the five dollars that his mother had sewed into his jacket. He quickly brought out his money and gave it to the man. He got on the train and went as far as Chicago—and then he had no more ticket! There he was, all alone in a big city in a strange land, not knowing what to do next, so he was sitting on the platform, crying. A gentleman walked by, talked to Joe, and recognized that he was speaking German, so he took the boy to a nearby saloon where he knew that the bartender-owner could speak German. Joe told his story, and the saloon keeper told him that he could stay there.

"'We'll write to your brothers,' he said, 'and keep you here until they send money so that you can get to where you want to go.'

"Joe stayed there and swept the floors and did a few odd jobs. In a week or two they had heard from his brothers, who sent enough money for his ticket, and he went on his way to Minnesota."

So the story ended well. One might question how a parent could send a 12-year-old child off by himself on such a long journey. Schooling ended for most European children at 12 years of age, and he would have been ready to look for a job. His parents no doubt felt that they were allowing him the opportunity to acquire his own land and thus better himself immensely. Land, which was valuable and difficult to acquire in his small native country, was readily available in the United States. With the short distances in Europe from one nation to another, his parents probably had no concept of the immense distance he would have to travel, across half of the continental United States. The five dollars that he was given for the trip was a lot of money, when one considers that $15, including board, was the year's wage in 1870 for Joseph Altmann's farm laborer.

BREY GRANDPARENTS

My grandfather, Alois Brey, owned a farm near Lafayette. Because it is known that he did not establish a homestead, he must have purchased his farm. He and Anna Altmann were married on January 9, 1881. Alois and Anna Brey were listed in the 1900 census of Lafayette Township in Nicollet County as having six children: Alouis (Louie) Peter (May, 1881), Joseph Henry (November, 1882), Anton (August, 1884), Franz (Francis or Frank) William (March, 1886), Theresa (November, 1887), and Mary (November, 1895) [Figure 1]. My father was born on March 22, 1886, the youngest of the four boys; the two girls came along later. Their father insisted that all of the boys help their mother with the housework. His attitude was unusual for a man of that time from a German background, but it no doubt explained why my father always seemed to be so comfortable, even enthusiastic, about pitching in to help with the household chores in our home.

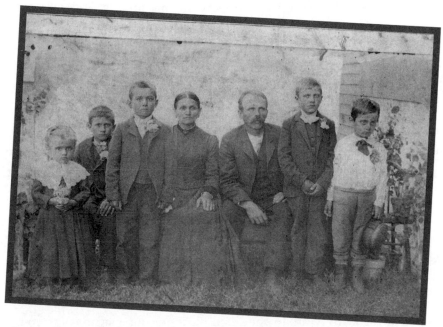

Fig. 1: *Photograph of the Brey family, circa 1895. Front row, from left, Theresa, Louie, Joseph, Anna, Alois, Anton, and Frank. Mary was born later.*

DISTRICT 69 ELEMENTARY SCHOOL

Not a great deal is known about my father's childhood and adolescence except that he did not talk very much and that he was a good student. For his grade school years, my father attended District 69 Elementary School in Lafayette Township of Nicollet County. German was spoken in the Brey home, and the children had their first exposure to English when they began to attend elementary school. (My mother's people, the Daub family, also spoke German in their home, and my mother also learned English beginning in the first grade.) My father believed that his lack of early exposure to English was a handicap, and he felt that he never became as articulate as he might otherwise have been. He must have learned to read and write German in school, because he was later excused from studying German when he enrolled in the University of Minnesota's pre-medicine program. Preserved in my family archives is a letter, written in German in Gothic script, which he wrote to his parents during his early years in practice in Wabasso.

TAPEWORM

We have never been sure why my father chose medicine as his profession, but his interest might have been stimulated by an incident that happened to his mother when he was a boy. An itinerant peddler who came around to the farm treated my grandmother for a tapeworm, which she expelled in due course. It was not uncommon in those days for people to obtain medical treatment in this way.

As a physician, my father treated a patient for a similar problem. After it was expelled, the tapeworm, a flatworm measuring 33 feet in length, was wound around a small wooden frame and immersed in alcohol or formaldehyde in a half-gallon glass canning jar. The specimen remained for many years in the linen closet of our bathroom at home, and I remember my father commenting on how important it was for the head of the tapeworm to be expelled along with the segments of its body. Otherwise, he said, the parasite would re-grow. It kept company with five small jars, each containing two small bits of tissue, the tonsils from four of my five siblings and myself. Ann recalls bringing the tapeworm to school for "show-and-tell," and I gained a good deal of respect from my friends when I brought them home to look at the entire collection. They were especially awed, of course, by the tapeworm.

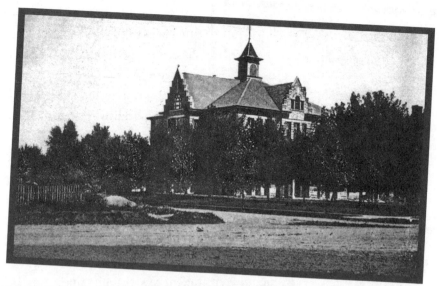

Fig. 2: *New Ulm High School, built in 1900, but no longer in existence.*

New Ulm High School

Because there was no high school in Lafayette, my father lived in a boarding house across the street from New Ulm High School [Figure 2], attending classes during the week and going home to the farm for the weekends and holidays. He played football, and a photograph of the players, which is no longer available, showed him standing in the front row, the tallest and largest member of the team.

The opportunity to attend high school was uncommon, especially for children who grew up on farms and small villages, and not many were so privileged. I believe he was the only one of his siblings to graduate from high school. This included his older brother Joseph, who went to an institution of higher learning and became a veterinarian without first attending high school. My mother, too, never attended high school but was able nevertheless to study nursing and become a registered nurse.

Among his high school texts were *First Lessons in Latin*, *Cicero: Selected Orations and Letters*, *Composition and Rhetoric*, *Introduction to English Literature*, and *A Brief Course in General Physics*. These books

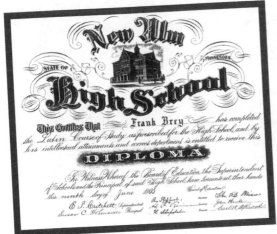

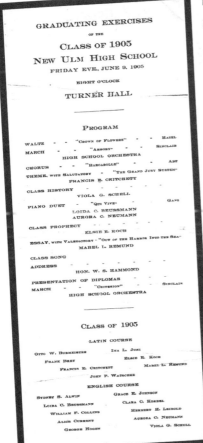

were preserved in the library of my family home. They must have served him well when he prepared for the entrance examination of the medical college at the University of Minnesota, which covered the following subjects: English composition, algebra, geometry, physics, United States history, physiology, and Latin (including Latin grammar and three books of Caesar). These seven requirements were far more stringent than those of most medical schools at that time. Frank Brey was awarded his diploma from New Ulm High School on June 9, 1905 [Figures 3 and 4].

HIS SIBLINGS' GAREER GHOICES

Each of Grandfather Brey's children, at 18 years of age, was given $2000 to use as he or she chose for education or career development. Two of the boys became farmers, with Louie on a farm of his own and Anton on the home place. Normally, the oldest son would have inherited the

(From Top to Bottom)

Fig. 3: *Frank Brey's diploma from New Ulm High School.*

Fig. 4: *Program and class listing for graduating exercises of the class of 1905, New Ulm High School, Friday, June 9, 1905. Frank Brey is listed as having taken the Latin Course.*

home place, but Uncle Louie was established on his own farm well before his parents were ready to leave their farm and retire to New Ulm. Both of the girls married farmers, and their money presumably served as their dowries.

Joseph was the only sibling who went on to receive a higher education. He first used his funds to establish a small general store near Lafayette, which he operated for a number of years while living at home. Unfortunately, there was a fire in the store, with loss of all of its contents and no insurance. The merchandise was replaced and he started over, but another fire occurred in the store, again with loss of all of its contents and no insurance. Joseph followed the example of his younger brother and decided to go to college. He passed the entrance examination and was accepted into veterinary school at almost 30 years of age without having attended high school. He left for his school in Missouri from Minneapolis in the autumn of 1910—my father had completed his medical school studies in the spring of that same year. Uncle Joe sometimes talked about his most lasting impression of Minneapolis: the streets of the city were so muddy after an unusually rainy season, he said, that the horses pulling buggies sank deep, up to their knees, in mud.

TEMPER, AND CHOOSING A CAREER

An anecdote told by Aunt Theresa Brey, Uncle Anton's wife, and repeated over the years throws additional light on my father's reasons for becoming a physician. In 1905, anyone with a high school diploma could teach the early grades in an elementary school without having received any special training as a teacher. Thus it came about that young Frank W. Brey, with his new diploma, proudly carrying his schoolbooks under his arm, applied for a job as an elementary school teacher in a one-room country school near Lafayette.

"You couldn't possibly teach these children," the principal told him. "You're much too young. Why, you look like a student yourself!"

"You know," said Aunt Theresa, "your dad had a temper in spite of being such a quiet person."

He came home, threw his books across the room, and announced, "That does it! I'm off to the university in the fall, and I'm going to be a doctor!"

REFERENCES

1. Folwell, William Watts. *A History of Minnesota*, vols I-IV. The Minnesota Historical Society, St. Paul, MN, published 1920, revised 1956.

2. Castle, Henry A. *Minnesota: Its Story and Biography*, vols I-III. The Lewis Publishing Co., Chicago and New York, 1915.

3. Clapesattle, Helen. *The Doctors Mayo*, The University of Minnesota Press, Minneapolis, 1941.

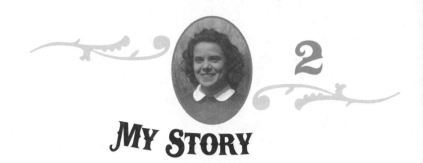

MY STORY

2

Not long ago I attended a pediatric hematology/oncology seminar at the Mayo Clinic. The subject that day was to be discussed by a young woman, and I was seated in the front of the room. While waiting to begin her presentation, because of a short delay while the viewing equipment was being set up, the young woman happened to glance at me.

"When did you graduate from medical school?" she asked me.

"Nineteen forty-six," I said.

"How many women were in your class?"

"Five."

"You helped lead the way for the rest of us," she said to me, "and we thank you."

I was deeply touched by her remark, and I realized then that perhaps some people might be interested in my story, too.

It seems obvious to me that my father's story as an old time family physician is important because he practiced medicine in a way that no longer exists. Although his story is only a small piece of the history of medicine, he was one of the country doctors who filled a unique and important place in his community during the early twentieth century. He was also my role model. Interwoven with the story of my father, who was an old time country doctor, is my own story of a woman who studied medicine and began practice at a time when very few women entered the profession. My father's story includes me up to the year of his death in 1940. My story starts at his death in 1940, when I was sixteen years old.

After I finished writing my father's biography, my daughter Alice, among others, began urging me to include something of myself, a woman who became a physician at a time when our numbers were relatively few. I resisted the idea, partly because I didn't think I was very interesting, and partly because some of the memories were painful. She presented me with James McBride's best selling book, *The Color Of Water* (G. K. Hall & Co., Thorndike, Maine, 1996), in which the author successfully entwines his own story as a black man with the story of his white mother.

A couple of reasons caused me to change my mind. First, I met several new friends, women physicians who were at the University of Minnesota Medical School or the Minneapolis General Hospital some years after my graduating date of 1946. One friend described her time in medical school as "four years of being treated like dirt." Consequently, she told me, she never cared to attend a class reunion, although she does continue to contribute toward a scholarship fund. Perhaps this attitude resulted from the "Herr Professor" style of teaching that was common among medical school professors in those days. I don't feel quite that strongly about my time in medical school, although I was sometimes "treated like dirt" during my pediatric residency.

Second, the position of women in medicine has changed remarkably since my school days and early years of practice. Many women are now training and working as physicians. In most medical school classes almost half—and in some more than half—of the students are currently women. As a result of affirmative action, it appears that women are sometimes even given preference for promotions and high level appointments. My friend had an opinion about that, too. "Since the profession of medicine no longer carries the prestige and good income that it once did," she said, "why not let women have it!"

One thing has not changed, however: women still bear the children and carry the major responsibility when it comes to raising them. I can only add that nothing is more rewarding than having a houseful of children to love and cherish with the help of a loving and devoted spouse.

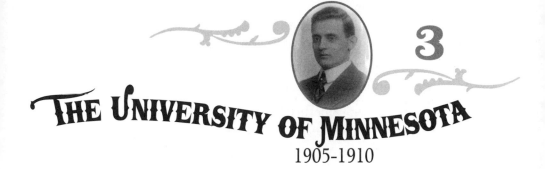

THE UNIVERSITY OF MINNESOTA
1905-1910

innesota's cold climate had attracted many patients with consumption (tuberculosis of the lung) during the period 1850 through 1870, but by 1880 the flow of consumptives was slowing and invalids from the East were more likely to head south or further west.[4] In the 1880s, diphtheria was the first cause of death, and tuberculosis the second cause of death in Minnesota. Other infectious diseases, especially typhoid fever and rabies, were serious public health problems in the state, as were also cholera and smallpox. Public health boards began to be established, at first in cities and later as permanent health agencies in local and state governments. Their purpose was mainly to regulate quarantine and general sanitation codes. Minnesota, the fourth state (after Massachusetts, California, and Virginia) to do so, established a State Board of Health in 1872.[5] The Minnesota Medical Society was founded in 1853, in what was still Minnesota Territory. Five years later, in 1858, Minnesota joined the union as a state. In 1869, the medical society, which had lapsed into inactivity, was reorganized and became the Minnesota State Medical Society.[5]

In 1905 Frank W. Brey began a five-year course at the University of Minnesota that would include one academic year, followed by four years of medicine. A six-year course, which required students to complete two academic years before starting the four-year medical course, had already been established but had not yet been made mandatory (it would become a requirement in 1906). Consequently, his was the last class that had both five-year and six-year students in the entering class.

When my father came to Minneapolis from the family farm near Lafayette in 1905, he must have been amazed and awed by the size of the city and its twin, St. Paul. The population of Minneapolis was almost 340,000, and the combined population of the two cities was close to 600,000. The population of Minnesota, according to the 1905 state census, was 1,979,912.

PIONEER PHYSICIANS

The first physician to practice in Minnesota was a military physician, Dr. Edward Purcell, who arrived with the first army contingent sent out to build Fort Snelling in 1819. Although there had been a few physicians among the fur traders and missionaries to the Indians, the first civilian physician to practice medicine in Minnesota was Dr. Christopher Carli, who settled in the Stillwater area near the Saint Croix River in 1841. St. Paul acquired its first physician, Dr. John Dewey, in 1847, and the first hospital in Minnesota, St. Joseph's Hospital in St. Paul, was opened in 1854.

THE UNIVERSITY OF MINNESOTA

The large university, located on the east bank of the great Mississippi River, with approximately 700 students enrolled, must have been equally impressive to young Frank Brey. By that time, eleven buildings had been built on the Minneapolis (main) campus of the university [Figures 5 and 6] and twelve on the St. Paul (agricultural) campus. Among the buildings on the main campus were Pillsbury Hall, Burton Hall, and Wesbrook Hall. The Psychology building and Shevlin Hall were added in 1906. Folwell Hall, the new main building for the College of Science, Literature and Arts was completed in 1907.

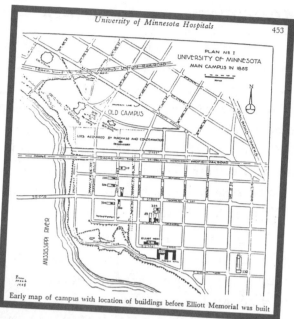

Early map of campus with location of buildings before Elliott Memorial was built

(From Top to Bottom)

Fig. 5: *Plan of the University of Minnesota main campus in 1885.*

Fig. 6: *The "gateway" to the main campus of the University of Minnesota at Fourteenth Street and University Avenue in 1905.*

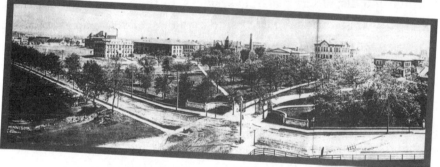

The University of Minnesota had been founded by the legislature in 1851, only two years after Minnesota became a territory in 1849, and seven years before it became a state in 1858. The original plan was for medicine to be one of the first five departments in the university (the others being science, literature, and arts; law; elementary education; and agriculture). In fact, the Department of Medicine [Appendix A] was not formally established until 1888, almost 40 years later. It was made up at first of three colleges: the College of Medicine and Surgery, the College of Homeopathic Medicine and Surgery, and the College of Dentistry. The College of Pharmacy became the fourth college in 1891.

HOMEOPATHY IN MINNESOTA

Homeopathy, considered a cult by traditional medicine, was a system of therapy developed by Samuel Hahnemann. According to his "law of similarities," or "principle of similars," diseases are treated with minute doses of drugs that can produce in healthy persons symptoms similar to those of the disease being treated—a sort of "fighting fire with fire" theory. Frequently a patient was better off than he or she would have been under treatment by the conventional medicine of the time because homeopathic doses were so small as to be without effect and nature was allowed to take its course.

The Minnesota Homeopathic Medical College became the university's College of Homeopathic Medicine and Surgery. As an autonomous unit within the Department of Medicine, it remained distinct from the College of Medicine and Surgery, with a separate faculty and separate hospital and dispensary teaching services for the homeopathy students. The two colleges, which existed side by side, had a similar curriculum because homeopathy accepted most teachings of conventional medicine. The curriculum of the homeopathic college did not include pathology or histology, however, and materia medica and therapeutics were taught in a very different way. Because homeopathy was respected by both patients and non-homeopathic physicians, it was able to demand autonomy and have its demand granted. By the middle of the nineteenth century, conventional medicine had lost a great deal of ground and had become quite unpopular because of its two chief forms of therapy: vigorous blood-letting and the administration of emetic and purgative drugs. Emetics induced vomiting and purgatives or cathartics caused evacuation of the bowels, both of which could and did make sick patients even sicker. Calomel, for example, was widely used; in addition to being a cathartic, the mercury it contained caused other toxic symptoms, including nerve damage. The treatment was often worse than the disease and, in some instances, even appeared to be a direct cause of death. Many physicians also questioned these methods of treatment. When Samuel Hahnemann proposed his less intensive therapeutic regimens in his book published in Germany in 1810, his ideas appealed to many people. It is not remarkable that a number of well-educated physicians switched to Hahnemann's more moderate methods, especially after his homeopathic treatment was shown to produce better survival rates among victims of cholera and typhoid fever epidemics.

The College of Homeopathic Medicine and Surgery enrollment was about one-fifth that of the College of Medicine and Surgery, and it graduated about five students each year. Gradual attrition occurred, however, as fewer and fewer students were attracted to homeopathy. In 1908 there were only three students enrolled in the college. No new students signed up in each of the ensuing years, and the school was closed in 1911. Only five percent of Minnesota physicians were homeopaths around the turn of the century, but I remember that a few well-regarded homeopathic physicians were still in active practice in Minneapolis when I enrolled in the University of Minnesota's medical school in 1943.

As a senior medical student in 1909-1910, my father must have been one of the first medical clerks in the University of Minnesota Hospitals. Senior medical students were called clerks. They were permitted, under the supervision of staff physicians, to examine patients, record their findings, and make suggestions for clinical management. The idea of clinical clerkships for medical students was a relatively new one that had been pioneered by William Osler at Johns Hopkins in 1895.

THE FLEXNER REPORT

In 1910 Abraham Flexner[6] reported to the Carnegie Foundation for the Advancement of Teaching on the status of 155 medical schools in the United States and Canada. His study was sponsored by the Foundation in response to a general impression that there was an excess of physicians and that most of them were poorly educated and poorly trained. The report concluded that there had been a huge overproduction of physicians during the preceding 25 years by a large number of inadequate schools that were being run purely for profit. The colleges and universities were failing to assume support of and responsibility for medical education. It urged that practical experience should supplement what was purely didactic teaching in many schools and recommended that hospitals as well as laboratories should be controlled by universities.

The University of Minnesota, which had been visited in May, 1909, received high praise for excellence in a number of areas. It was one of only 16 of the 155 institutions that required two years of college work for entrance, including science and a modern language. It was commended for being "perhaps the first state in the Union" to consolidate medical education (except for osteopathy, which was not included in Minnesota's consolidation) within a single institution. It had "by statesmanlike action got rid of all other medical schools in the state," thus placing medical education "in the hands of" the university. It was the only medical school in Minnesota, and also the only medical school in the Northwest between Milwaukee and Seattle.

Flexner noted that for a population of almost two million, there were 2204 physicians in the state, a ratio of one physician per 981 persons. There were 174 students enrolled in the medical school, 83 percent of them from Minnesota. The teaching staff consisted of 49 professors and 71 others, to a total of 120. The annual budget was $71,336, of which $16,546 came from fees and the rest from a state appropriation. Flexner stated that the medical school in Minneapolis must help supply physicians for North and South Dakota and Montana. (These states still did not have four-year medical schools when I was a medical student at the University of Minnesota in 1943-1946, hence students from those states were in classes with me.)

Flexner commended the University of Minnesota College of Medicine and Surgery for its "excellent, exceedingly attractive, and well organized laboratories" and for its full time teachers, with salaried chiefs of medicine and surgery. So impressed was Flexner by the school's laboratories that he referred to them in the general discussion section of his report as "admirable" and complimented the Canadian schools, McGill and Toronto, by saying that "in point of laboratory equipment, they equal Minnesota." The importance of its location in the largest community in the state (the combined Minneapolis-St. Paul population was 552,211), so that the entire four-year course could be completed in one institution, was remarked upon. Recent reorganization of the clinical teaching and the dispensary received favorable comment. The only fault found was in the lack of a teaching hospital, which was already being built. Elliot Memorial Hospital would be completed in 1911. Flexner also commended the state board, noting that it had not only cooperated with the University in establishing medical standards, but that it also required any practitioner who was trained elsewhere to have a similar premedical and professional education.

FRANK W. BREY

When my father entered the medical school, there were four buildings in use on the medical campus, and another was added during his time as a student. Cyrus Northrop (1884-1910), the much-loved "prexy" who was the University's second president, remained in this position throughout my father's time at the University. Parks Ritchie (1897-1906), the second dean of the medical school, resigned from the deanship in 1906 but remained on the faculty as professor of obstetrics. He was replaced by Frank F. Wesbrook (1906-1913), professor of pathology and bacteriology, who became the first full-time dean of the medical school.

FIRST YEAR

A copy of my father's academic transcript, obtained from the office of the Registrar, shows that his first year (1905-1906) was spent in the College of Science, Literature and the Arts [Figure 7]. He received P (passing) grades for two semesters each of mathematics, military drill, gymnasium, animal biology, and chemistry, and one semester of rhetoric. (His rhetoric teacher was probably Maria Sanford. The women's dormitory in which I lived during my first year in the University's undergraduate school was named for her.) He was excused from what otherwise would have been two semesters of German.

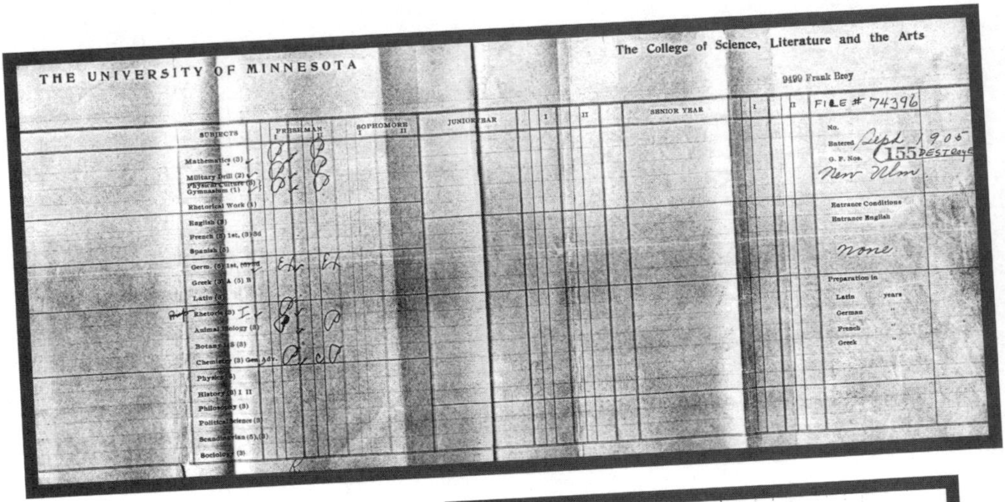

THE UNIVERSITY OF MINNESOTA

The College of Science, Literature and the Arts

9490 Frank Brey

FILE # 74396

Entered Sept 1905

New Ulm

Entrance Conditions

Entrance English

none

SUBJECTS	FRESHMAN I	FRESHMAN II
Mathematics (3)	G	G
Military Drill (2)	G	G
Physical Culture (3) Gymnasium (1)	G	P
Rhetorical Work (1)		
English (3)		
French (3) 1st, (3) 2d		
Spanish (3)		
Germ. (3) 1st	Ex	Ex
Greek (3) A (5) B		
Latin (3)		
Rhetoric (3)	G	P
Animal Biology (3)		
Botany (3)		
Chemistry (3) Gen. Adv.	G	P
Physics (3)		
History (3) I II		
Philosophy (3)		
Political Science (3)		
Scandinavian (5), (3)		
Sociology (3)		

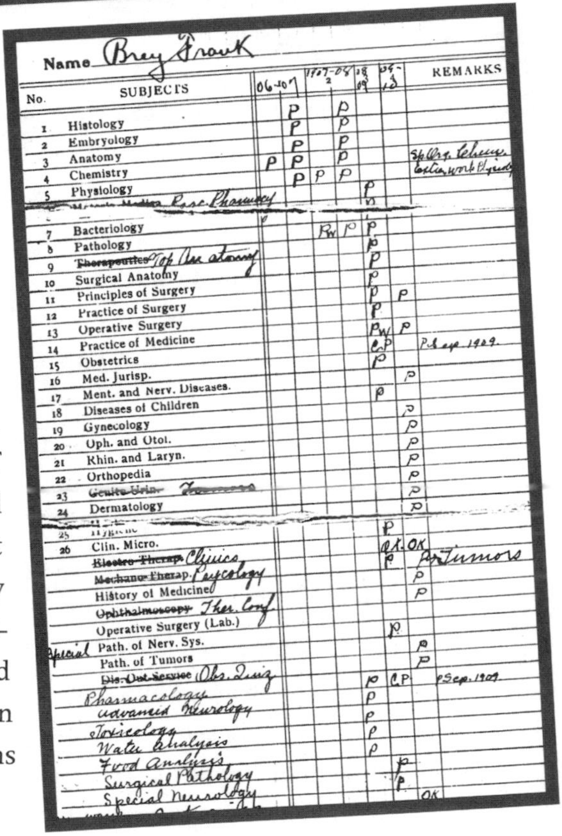

Name Brey Frank

No.	SUBJECTS	06-07	1907-08	08-09	09-10	REMARKS
1	Histology		P	P		
2	Embryology		P	P		
3	Anatomy		P	P		
4	Chemistry	P	P	P		
5	Physiology		P P	P	P	
7	Bacteriology			Pw P	P	
8	Pathology				P	
9	Top. Anatomy				P	
10	Surgical Anatomy				P	
11	Principles of Surgery				P	P
12	Practice of Surgery				P	
13	Operative Surgery				Pw	P
14	Practice of Medicine				CP	P Sep. 1909
15	Obstetrics				P	
16	Med. Jurisp.					P
17	Ment. and Nerv. Diseases				P	
18	Diseases of Children					P
19	Gynecology					P
20	Oph. and Otol.					P
21	Rhin. and Laryn.					P
22	Orthopedia					P
23	Tumors					P
24	Dermatology					P
26	Clin. Micro.				P	

MEDICAL SCHOOL

His academic transcript for the next four years [Figure 8] shows that they were spent in the College of Medicine and Surgery, again with passing grades in all subjects [Table 1]. From its beginning, the medical school had emphasized the study of pathology and had insisted that every medical student learn to perform an autopsy correctly. Students participated in autopsies in the "dead house" under the supervision of the pathologist who was assigned to the case.

(From Top to Bottom)

Fig. 7: *Frank Brey's academic transcript from the College of Science, Literature and the Arts, 1905-1906.*

Fig. 8: *Frank Brey's academic transcript from the College of Medicine and Surgery, 1906-1910.*

(From Top to Bottom)

Fig. 9: *Small group of sophomore anatomy students assigned to dissect one cadaver. They are shown gowned, capped, and gloved, along with the cadaver, who is also gowned, capped, and perhaps gloved. My father stands at the far right.*

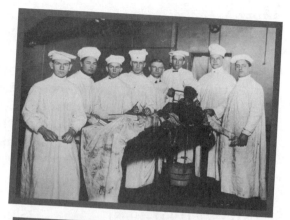

Fig. 10: *Probably the entire class of sophomore anatomy students. My father is the first student on the left in the second row.*

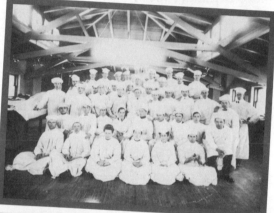

Fig. 11: *Probably the entire medical school class of 1910. Their formal dress most likely indicates that they were engaged in their clinical services, circa 1908-1910. My father is the third student from the left in the third row.*

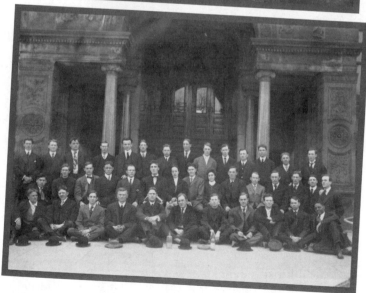

TABLE 1. *Medical student Frank W. Brey's curriculum for his four years at the University of Minnesota Medical School (1906-1910).*

FIRST YEAR (1906–1907)
Histology
Embryology
Anatomy
Chemistry
Physiology
Extra work in physiology

SECOND YEAR (1907–1908)
Histology
Embryology and Sense Organs
Anatomy
Chemistry (Toxicology, Water, Food Analysis, Organic Chemistry)
Physiology
Pharmacology
Toxicology
Water Analysis
Food Analysis
Advanced Neurology

THIRD YEAR (1908–1909)
Pharmacology and Therapeutics
Pathology and Bacteriology (Special)
Surgical Anatomy
Principles of Surgery
Practice of Surgery
Operative Surgery
Practice of Medicine (Lectures)
Obstetrics
Medical Jurisprudence
Pediatrics

Third year (continued)
Pharmacology—Practical Pharmacy
Clinical Microscopy
Clinics
Psychology
Special Pathology of the Nervous System
Special Neurology
Surgical Pathology
Topographical Anatomy

FOURTH YEAR (1909–1910)
Therapeutic Conference
Practice of Surgery
Tumors
Operative Surgery
Practice of Medicine
Obstetrics
Mental and Nervous Diseases
Gynecology
Ophthalmology and Otology (Eye and Ear)
Rhinology and Laryngology (Nose and Throat)
Orthopedics
Clinical Microscopy
Dematology
Hygiene
History of Medicine
Pathology of Tumors
Clinics (Dispensary Service)
Autopsies

A pair of photographs found among my father's papers appear to be from anatomy class. One, which has a macabre theme, shows a small dissection group in anatomy class [Figure 9]. The students, wearing gowns, caps, and gloves, are shown with a cadaver, which is propped up in a sitting position and also adorned with a cap. The other, dated February 4, 1907, and labeled "sophomore medic" and "Metropolitan Theater," appears to include the entire sophomore anatomy class [Figure 10]. Pencilled notations on the second photograph—"Babe-Frank...ginger ale, high-balls, bourbon...walk home...time, place, & girl"—seem to indicate that a party is being planned. A third, considerably more formal photograph [Figure 11], was probably taken a couple of years later. That the men students are dressed in shirts and ties most likely indicates that the students were seeing patients in a clinical setting.

TEXTBOOKS

A number of my father's medical textbooks, related to the subjects listed above, remain in the library of my family home [Table 2]. One textbook, the sixth edition of May's *Manual of the Diseases of the Eye,* is especially interesting to me because I studied May's eighteenth edition of the same textbook (published, 1943) for my course in ophthalmology when I was in medical school.

THE COST OF MEDICAL EDUCATION

His academic transcript shows the fees that were paid for the four years of medical school [Figure 12], each payment having been made "by cash," to a total of $515 for eight semesters, including microscope fees for four of the semesters. He was required to furnish his own microscope, a monocular instrument that was still in his possession at the time of his death. Additional expenses, not included in the $515 paid for tuition, were the fees for his first academic year and the cost of textbooks, room, board, and clothing.

He roomed, as did most of he students, in various houses, and at one time, according to an address written beneath his name in one of

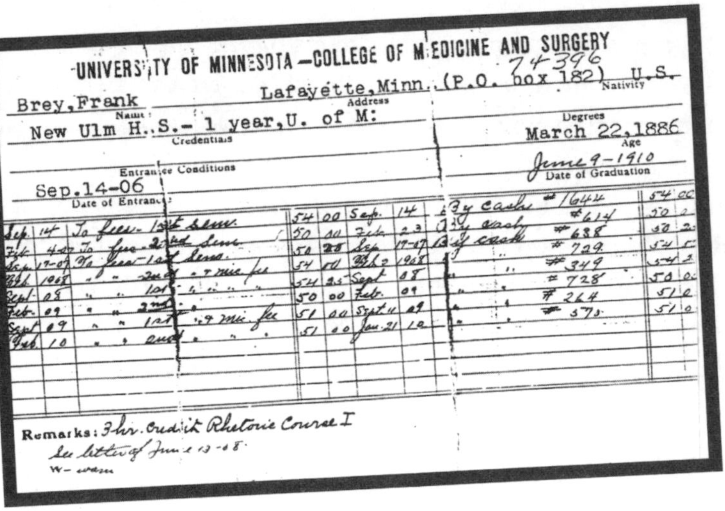

UNIVERSITY OF MINNESOTA—COLLEGE OF MEDICINE AND SURGERY

74396

Brey, Frank — Name

Lafayette, Minn. (P.O. box 182) — Address

U.S. — Nativity

New Ulm H. S.- 1 year, U. of M: — Credentials

Degrees

March 22, 1886 — Age

Entrance Conditions

June 9-1910 — Date of Graduation

Sep. 14-06 — Date of Entrance

Remarks: 3 hr. Credit Rhetoric Course I

Fig. 12: *Record of tuition payments by Frank Brey to the College of Medicine and Surgery, 1906-1910.*

TABLE 2. *Partial list of medical textbooks from Dr. Frank W. Brey's student days. These books and others are still on the shelves at the Brey family home*

Hecktoen, Ludvig, and Riesman, David. *An American Text-Book of Pathology: for the Use of Students and Practitioners of Medicine and Surgery*. W.B. Saunders & Co., Philadelphia, 1902.

Sollmann, Torald. *A Text-Book of Pharmacology and Some Allied Sciences (Therapeutics, Materia Medica, Pharmacy, Prescription Writing, Toxicology, etc.): Together with Outlines for Laboratory Work, Solubility and Dose Tables, etc., 2nd ed.* W. B. Saunders & Co., Philadelphia, 1906.

Manual of Therapeutics. Parke Davis & Co., Detroit, Michigan, 1909.

Anders, James M. *A Text-Book of the Practice of Medicine, 9th Ed.* W. B. Saunders & Co., Philadetphia, 1909.

Rose, William, and Carless, Albert. *A Manual of Surgery: for Students and Practitioners, 7th ed.* William Wood & Co., New York, 1908.

Lexer, Ehrich, edited by Bevan, Arthur Dean, translated by Lewis, Dean. *General Surgery: a Presentation of the Scientific Principles upon Which the Practice of Modern Surgery is Based, 2nd Ed.* D. Appleton & Co., New York, 1908

Ashton, William Easterlly. *A Text-Book on the Practice of Gynecology: for Practitioners and Students, 3rd ed.* W. B. Saunders & Co., Philadelphia, 1908.

May Charles H. *Manual of the Diseases of the Eye: for Students and General Practitioners, 6th ed.* William Wood & Co., New York, 1909.

his texts titled *A Manual of Surgery* [Table 2], he resided at 220 Church Street Southeast in Minneapolis. He tended the furnace to partially pay for his room and board in at least one of the rooming houses. During his senior year of medical school he stayed in the College Inn Hotel on Fourth Street Southeast, which at that time was considered to be quite an elegant residence. My sister Ann remembers that he showed us children the building on a nostalgic visit to Minneapolis in which we toured the University of Minnesota campus. One might speculate that the $2000 allotted him by his father appeared to be nicely covering his expenses, with some left over, and perhaps he had decided to "treat" himself in that final medical school year.

An approximation of how expensive a medical education in the upper midwest was can be found in the Flexner report. A six-year course (two years of college followed by four years of medicine) at the University of Michigan in Ann Arbor cost $1466 for tuition fees, room, and board in 1909. A similar program at Minnesota, according to Flexner, would cost "very little more."

ALPHA KAPPA KAPPA

My father joined the Psi chapter of Alpha Kappa Kappa (AKK), a professional medical fraternity that had been instituted in Minnesota in 1898. A fraternity house is pictured in *The Gopher*, the Minnesota yearbook for 1910. No address is given, however, and it is not known whether he ever lived there. He is listed in the fraternity's catalogue as being a member of the class of 1910, as is Monte Charles Piper, who practiced after graduation in Lamberton, Minnesota, and later joined the staff of the Mayo Clinic. Otto John Seifert of New Ulm is listed as a member of the class of 1912. They were good friends throughout my father's lifetime.

GRADUATION AND LICENSURE

Frank W. Brey was awarded the Doctor of Medicine degree from the College of Medicine and Surgery at the University of Minnesota on June

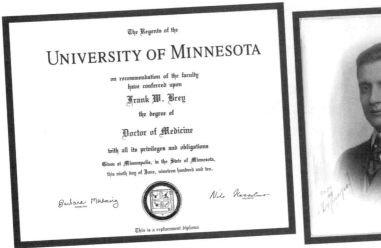

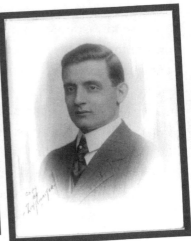

(From Left to Right)

Fig 13: *Doctor of Medicine diploma awarded by the University of Minnesota to Frank W. Brey on June 9, 1910.*

Fig. 14: *Formal graduation photograph of Frank W. Brey, M.D.*

9, 1910 [Figure 13]. The description under his photograph in the 1910 yearbook [Figure 14] states, "As a freshman, he was noted as an after-dinner speaker." The formal invitation to the graduation ceremony identifies him as a member of the Social Committee for the occasion [Figure 15 a-d]. Because he had the reputation of being extremely quiet and shy at that time of his life, my family has always considered these remarks to have been a bit of mild teasing.

Students who had completed their schooling and received their Doctor of Medicine degrees were considered to be fully qualified in medicine and could begin practice immediately. Internship was not required for the M.D. degree, and only the few who had decided to specialize would stay on for further training. In 1911, a year later, the University of Minnesota would begin awarding Bachelor of Medicine (M.B.) degrees at graduation, and M.D. degrees only after a year of internship was completed. (When I graduated from the University of Minnesota Medical School in 1946, this system was still in place.) Frank W. Brey had already passed the basic science examination and was in possession

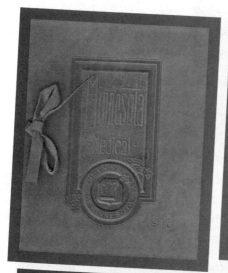

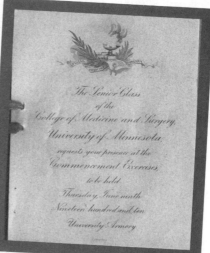

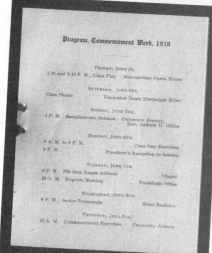

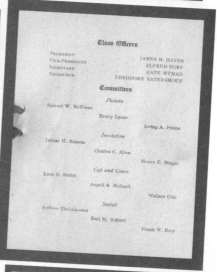

(From Top to Bottom)

Fig. 15a-d: *Invitation to the commencement exercises of the College of Medicine and Surgery, University of Minnesota, 1910. Frank W. Brey is listed as a member of the Social Committee.*

Fig. 16: *Minnesota Medical License for 1940, the final year of Frank W. Brey's life.*

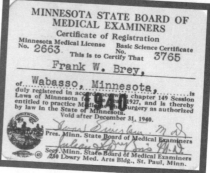

of Basic Science Certificate number 3765. He received, by examination, Minnesota Medical License number 2663 from the Minnesota State Board of Medical Examiners on June 29, 1910 [Figure 16].

Dr. Brey was ready to begin seeing patients [Appendix B].

REFERENCES

4. Meyers, J. Arthur. *Masters of Medicine: An Historical Sketch of the College of Medical Sciences, University of Minnesota 1888-1966.* Warren H. Green, Inc., St. Louis, Missouri, 1968.

5. Wilson, Leonard G. *Medical Revolution in Minnesota: A History of the University of Minnesota Medical School.* Midewiwin Press, St. Paul, MN, 1989.

6. Flexner, Abraham. *Medical Educaton in the United States and Canada: A Report to the Carnegie Foundation for the Advancement of Teaching* with an Introduction by Henry D. Pritchett. D. B. Updike, the Merrymount Press, Boston, 1910.

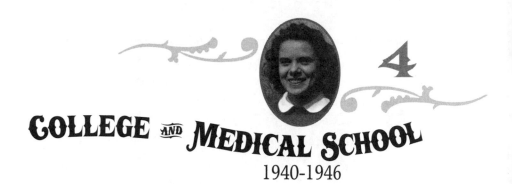

COLLEGE AND MEDICAL SCHOOL
1940-1946

My life changed completely in 1940. I turned sixteen in February, my father died in June, and I became a freshman at the University of Minnesota in September. Starting at five years of age, I had told my parents that I wanted to become a doctor. This concerned my mother, who felt that I should be discouraged from such an ambition. My father told her not to discourage me, however, because by the time I was ready for medical school women would be more readily accepted into the profession. There was one woman in his medical school class and there were a few in some of the other classes. "Hens, we called them," he said, "hen medics."

COLLEGE 1940~1943

Our neighbors and good friends, John and Charlotte Bradish, along with their daughter Elaine, gave me a ride to the freshman girls' dormitory, Sanford Hall, and helped us move in. Elaine and I had been friends since we were babies and now we were roommates. Sanford Hall, by the way, was named for Maria Sanford, a distinguished professor of English who was on the university staff when my father was a student; she might have been one of his teachers. I enrolled in the College of Science, Literature, and Arts (SLA) with a major in pre-medicine, and Elaine enrolled in the General College.

College was both frightening and exhilarating for me. For one thing, very few young persons from Wabasso had attended college. For another, I was well aware of my youth and inexperience and the deficits in my education. I soon observed that the students coming from Minneapolis schools were much better prepared than I was. For example, many of them coasted through easily, especially in chemistry and physics classes, because they had already learned the material in high school. Wabasso schools offered no language courses except for English, so I began studying German, which was required for admission to medical school. I also enrolled in beginning algebra and trigonometry courses. I was worried that I might not make it in college, and at the same time I was excited and full of enthusiasm because of the opportunity to explore a new world and learn new things.

I lived in Sanford Hall as a freshman, and in Comstock Hall during my sophomore and junior years. The Second World War began in 1941 while I was living in Comstock Hall during my second year of college; I remember sitting in my room at my desk, studying, when I heard the announcement that we were at war. Among the girls who lived on my floor in the dormitory were several advanced students from the Mesabi Iron Range: Helen Golden, Audrey Arcola, and Marg and Busy Loye. Northern Minnesota was very prosperous at that time because the iron mines were still producing high quality ore, and the communities gave generous support to their schools. The Northern high schools and community colleges offered an excellent education, and my friends from the North, who were bright girls, were well grounded in the basic subjects. Without their kind help I surely would have floundered; with their help I kept my head above water and made good enough grades to get into medical school at 19 years of age, after three years of college. It was usual then to be admitted to medical school after three years of pre-medicine.

MEDICAL SCHOOL 1943-1946

I started medical school in 1943, two years after the United States had entered the Second World War in 1941. Because physicians were needed for the military services, the University of Minnesota Medical School, which ran on a quarter system along with the rest of the university, had accelerated its classes by deleting the summer vacation. In this way the curriculum was preserved intact. Our class began in April instead of in September, and the men in the class, except for a few who had medical problems, were inducted into either the Army or the Navy. From then on the men attended classes in uniform and received military training during the brief vacations between school quarters. They marched to school in formation and lived in barracks for the first two years. After that they no longer marched to school and were not restricted as to where they could live. When we started seeing patients in the clinical years, the third and fourth years of medical school, patients loved having these young service men help care for them. This was especially obvious with the children on the pediatric wards. Their eyes would light up and their faces would shine when they saw a real live uniformed soldier or sailor appear as their student doctor. Tuition, books, clothing, board, and room were furnished for my classmates, and they each received the pay of a private first class in the Army or its equivalent for those in the Navy. We women received no financial assistance. Tuition at the University of Minnesota was, however, very minimal. I had paid $35 each quarter while in undergraduate school, and my tuition was increased to $86 dollars per quarter for medical school.

WEST RIVER ROAD

I lived in Comstock Hall for my first year of medical school and then moved with my sisters Ann and Virginia to a rooming house on West River Road, about a half-mile from the medical campus. For awhile we had the entire third floor, with a kitchen and our own bathroom. West River Road, on the west bank of the Mississippi River, was an elegant location. Next door to our rooming house was the Alpha Kappa Kappa medical fraternity house—this was the fraternity to which my father had belonged many years earlier. I enjoyed the beautiful view of the river as I walked to school in the mornings and home in the evenings. When I began dating Fran, he and I spent many evenings along the

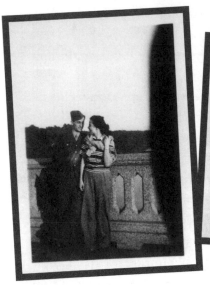
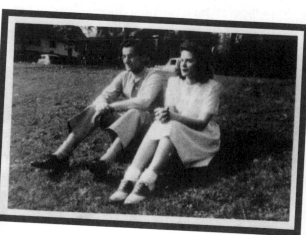

(From Left To Right)
Fig. 17: *Terry and Fran at the Lake Street Bridge in Minneapolis.*
Fig. 18: *Terry and Fran relaxing along West River Road.*

river bank [Figures 17 and 18]. Across the river was a park with an out-door ice rink, where we occasionally skated in winter.

Ann was enrolled at the University of Minnesota in a home economics program. Virginia graduated from a local Minneapolis high school and enrolled in a nursing program at St. Catherine's College nearby. At this time my brother Al was in the Navy Air Corps learning to be a pilot, and the two younger siblings, Paul and Justine, were in boarding school. My mother had enrolled in a refresher nursing course at the University of Minnesota and was living at a separate boarding house. She later accepted a position as a psychiatric nurse at the St. Cloud State Hospital.

TEACHERS

The University of Minnesota Medical School had an outstanding faculty that included a number of department chairmen who were nationally and internationally recognized. Among them were Elexious

T. Bell, who wrote the definitive textbook of pathology and was acclaimed as a teacher; Maurice B. Visscher, known for his studies in cardiovascular physiology and for promoting the use of animals in research; Owen H. Wangensteen, a famous surgeon whose best known work was on intestinal obstruction; Cecil J. Watson, an internist who studied the liver and the chemistry of bile; and Irvine McQuarrie, a pediatric endocrinologist whose residency program produced many pediatric departmental chairmen across the nation. George E. Fahr, who was chairman of internal medicine at the Minneapolis General Hospital was also one of our important teachers. He had studied in Germany with Einthoven, the inventor of the electrocardiograph, and was known informally by the students as "God." The students called his assistant "Jesus Christ." After completing our first two years studying the basic sciences, we were introduced to clinical medicine in clinical clerkships. We wore short white coats on the wards and when seeing our patients, and we were called clerks. We were assigned to rotations in Minneapolis General Hospital as well as in the University of Minnesota Hospitals.

CLASSMATES

Of 104 students in the entering freshman class, five of us were women: Ethel Erickson, Christine Furman, Jane Gumprecht, Mary Jane Jensen, and myself. Audrey Arcola, who started with us, dropped out

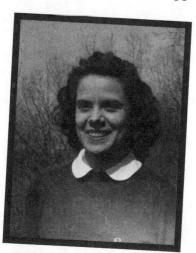

Fig. 19: *Terry as a first year medical student at the University of Minnesota.*

after being ill for six weeks with infectious mononucleosis. I worried at first about whether I could compete academically, but we women encouraged each other and I found that I could do the work. I joined Alpha Epsilon Iota medical sorority [Figure 19], which included women in the upper classes and functioned as a support group for all of the women in medical school.

Except for the other women in my class and Fran's fraternity brothers, I did not get to know many of my classmates very well. A classmate who later became famous as the first person to perform a bone marrow transplant was Bob Good; he and I both dropped out after our sophomore year and we both resumed classes in our junior year at the same time. While I earned money to pay my tuition, however, Bob earned a Ph.D. in anatomy. His situation was unusual in that his medical school tuition was paid from a scholarship at a time when scholarships were extremely rare and very few students were fortunate enough to hold one. Bob's mother was a widowed schoolteacher who was raising several sons. I had first known him in physical chemistry class, where he sat next to me at his laboratory microscope. Bob always blew in like a breath of fresh air, full of enthusiasm and ready for class, after finishing work at his night job. He was already on his way to medical and scientific excellence, and it's not surprising that he had been identified by his teachers as someone to watch.

RESENTMENT

Some of the men in my class (some of the men on the faculty, too) resented the presence of women students. My fellow students made comments such as, "You took a place that should have been filled by a man. You'll only get married, have children, and end up by never practicing medicine!" Sometimes the remarks were said in an unpleasant, spiteful tone, but at other times they were spoken sadly, with a shake of the head, as if meant only "for your own good." I started dating Fran, who later became and still is my husband, during my freshman year in medical school, and this probably protected me in a major way from slurs and worse. He was a member of Phi Chi medical fraternity, and I could count on him as well as his fraternity brothers for help if needed.

EMPLOYMENT

After my second year of medical school I dropped out for an academic year to work full time and help out my family's finances by earning enough money for my last two years' tuition. Since my mother had four children younger than I to feed, clothe, and educate, I felt that I should help out by at least partially supporting myself. (Even my undergraduate tuition of $35 per quarter and medical school tuition of $86 per quarter strained our family budget.) These were the World War II years, and because so many people had left for the front, there were a good many employment opportunities. I joined the Department of Pharmacology, with Raymond N. Bieter, M.D., as chairman and Harold N. Wright, Ph.D., as vice-chairman. During that year, I was privileged to become an author of my very first scientific paper.[7] My contribution to the article consisted of caring for the cotton rats that were the experimental subjects, and inclusion of my name as an author was a kind gesture on the part of the pharmacology staff. This accomplishment stimulated my interest in academic medicine, however, and probably explains my pursuit of an academic career when the opportunity arose much later in my life. I was allowed to take the pharmacology course along with my fellow classmates, and, with only one subject to study, I did well in the course. After completing my year off, which actually amounted to nine months because of the accelerated medical school curriculum, I joined the next class and became a junior medical student. That year off must have helped me to mature, because my grades improved during my junior and senior years. I continued to work part time for the Department of Pharmacology, and one year I earned $1100. I was outraged that I had to pay income tax that year on such a small amount! It wasn't enough to cover my room and board, so it didn't seem fair that I should have to pay part of it to the government!

AN OVERHEARD CONVERSATION

In order to get away from my rooming house for a quiet atmosphere, I often went to the university library to study. Sometimes Fran went with me and we had a "study date." Also, I occasionally studied in the Department of Pharmacology conference room during the evening hours or on weekends. One Saturday afternoon, when I was studying alone in the Department of Pharmacology, I overheard a conversation from the office down the hall that was not meant for my ears. Dr. Bieter was in the process of quietly firing his head technician. "I'm sorry about this," he said to the man, "but you know the reason why I can't keep you on." Later I learned that the man owned a tavern, and in the evenings and weekends he was dispensing drinks made with ethanol stolen from the Department. Ethanol is pure, colorless ethyl or grain alcohol; cocktails made from it no doubt carry a very effective punch. I realized that it was important for Dr. Bieter to handle the matter quietly because, even though only the technician was guilty of criminal activity, the matter would have reflected badly on both the Department and the University.

SKELETON

My skeleton was given to me by Dr. Wright, during my year of full time work in the Department of Pharmacology. It was the torso of a human skeleton that had previously been used to teach medical students how to do a lumbar puncture (insert a needle between the vertebrae into the spinal canal in order to extract spinal fluid for analysis or instill a drug such as a spinal anesthetic). It no doubt had come from one of the bodies used for anatomical dissection in the gross anatomy laboratory. Most of such specimens came from the bodies of local derelicts who had died without family or friends, or individuals who had donated their bodies to the University for scientific use. I had seen pictures of old time physicians with skeletons in their offices, and I thought that a skeleton would add a professional look to my office when the time came for me to start practice. It did not occur to me that getting rid of it might be a problem some day. For a while it hung in the clothes closet in our apartment in the rooming house on West River Road. Surprisingly, our landlady never objected to the skeleton's presence. More about the skeleton later.

WORLD WAR II ENDED

We were aware of food rationing and gas rationing (none of us had automobiles), but mainly we were too busy to think much about the ongoing war. Both of my brothers were too young to be actually engaged in the fighting. Al spent two years training to be a Navy pilot and graduated just as the war ended. Paul, who was younger, served two years in the Army after the war was over. All of the men in Fran's family except his dad were in the service. His sister Bea's husband, Tony, was injured, but fortunately there were no deaths among his close relatives.

VJ DAY AND THAT PHOTO

The war was finally over on VJ Day (Victory in Japan Day), August 14, 1945. A famous photo of a sailor celebrating the end of the war by kissing a nurse in Times Square, taken by a photographer for Life magazine, continues to be shown in newspapers and magazines on every anniversary of that date. I hate that photo! It reminds me of what happened to me on VJ Day. Around nine o'clock at night I was waiting at a bus stop one block from the Minneapolis General Hospital, on my way home after finishing my work on a clinical clerkship there. I was nervous because it was dark and the hospital was located in a bad part of town. (Most municipal hospitals for indigent patients are located in high crime areas.) I could hear bells and sirens celebrating the end of the war coming from the center of Minneapolis, a few blocks away, but there seemed to be no one on my street. Then suddenly, out of nowhere, a man came and tried to grab me. He was probably drunk and harmless, but he frightened me. I struggled free and ran, crying, back to the hospital, where I spent the rest of the night in the students' call room. Interestingly, it never occurred to me to report the incident to the hospital authorities or to the police. Now when I hear that photo described as "romantic," I tell myself, "I'll bet that nurse didn't think it was 'romantic'—but at least, in her case, there were lots of people around!"

WHAT I LEARNED IN MEDICAL SCHOOL

In my four years of medical school, I learned a lot about the treatment of diseases and how to deal with patients. The main things I learned, however, were to "do my work, mind my own business, and keep my mouth shut!"

REFERENCE

7. Wright, H. N., Litchfield, J. T., Jr., Brey, T. E., Cranston, E. M., Cuckler, A. C., Bieter, R. N. Chemotherapeutic activity of cyanines and related compounds in filariasis in the cotton rat. *Ann NY Acad Sc* 50:109-114, 1948.

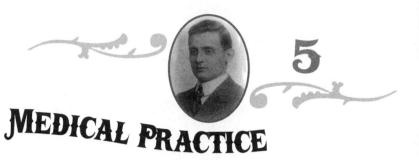

MEDICAL PRACTICE

THE EARLY YEARS
1910-1925

he first major obstacle to successful surgery had been solved by the introduction of general anesthesia around the time of the Civil War. By the end of the nineteenth century, methods of controlling infection became available, and the second major obstacle to surgical advance was overcome. Antisepsis, which was introduced to Minnesota in the early 1880's, preceded the development of several important surgical techniques. The first gall bladder operation in the state was performed by a St. Paul surgeon in 1886 and the first appendectomy by another St. Paul surgeon in 1887. Tenderness at McBurney's point, an important diagnostic finding in appendicitis, and McBurney's incision, a surgical approach for removing an inflamed appendix, were described in 1889 and 1894, respectively, by Charles McBurney in New York. Antisepsis, in which microorganisms were killed, was gradually replaced by asepsis, in which microorganisms were kept out of a sterile operating field. Complete asepsis became possible after surgical gloves, first used in Johns Hopkins Hospital in Baltimore in 1889, became generally available.

The reason why young Dr. Frank W. Brey chose to begin practicing medicine in the tiny town of Wabasso, Minnesota, which had a population of 343 in 1910 (Table 3), is not known. It is clear, however, that he

TABLE 3. *Population figures for Wabasso Village, Vail Township, and Redwood County, 1865-1940.*

Date	Wabasso Village	Vail Township	Redwood County
1865[1]	--	--	--
1870	--	--	869 or 1829
1880[2]	--	61	3375 or 5375
1890	--	213	9386
1900[3]	178	497	17261
1910	343	553	
1920	459	553	
1930	482	564	
1940	604	546	

[1] Redwood County was created by the Minnesota legislature on February 6, 1862, but because the act was not ratified by popular vote, it did not legally become a county until February 23, 1865, when the county's borders were re-established by the legislature.

[2] Vail Township was established in 1880.

[3] Wabasso Village came into existence in 1900.

intended to do his best to serve the people of the town and outlying areas. "He always came," said Loren Beran as he reminisced about how Dr. Brey came to their home one night by horse and buggy. "The doctor arrived about ten o'clock in the evening, in the pouring rain, with his black bag," said Loren. "He had a very quiet voice and a soothing manner. He always came."

Five doctors had practiced in Wabasso before my father arrived, but none of them stayed very long: Dr. Herman E. Lucas, Dr. A. G. Chadbourn, Dr. E. W. Gag, Dr. Schneider, and Dr. G. L. Gossle. A sixth doctor, Dr. M. G. Bickford, came to town in 1910, the same year my father arrived, and continued to practice in Wabasso until he left in 1913. These practitioners are listed in Arnold J. Bauer's book, *The Story of Wabasso*, published in 1934. Mr. Bauer included his opinion of Dr. Brey: "He has been very successful in his profession here and his work has given general satisfaction. He has an office located on Main Street."

WABASSO

Like the other frontier towns of central Redwood County, Wabasso was a "railroad town," one of a series of four small prairie towns strung slant-wise across the center of Redwood County. It was founded by a subsidiary of the Chicago and Northwestern Railroad Company at the turn of the century to carry away the grain grown in the black loam of this fertile and highly productive agricultural area. Wheat was the principal export, and corn was second. A grain elevator was often the first building built in these towns, sometimes even before the railroad was in place.

The railroad land company bought property in the center of Redwood County, which was almost empty except for farms like my great-grandfather Daub's homestead. The railroad route included not only land for the tracks, railroad yards, and depot, but also townsites along the route. The towns were spaced at intervals so that every farmer in the area could, by traveling not more than half a day in each direction, carry grain by wagon to grain elevators. Thus, the farmer would not have to be away from home overnight. The railroad companies platted the town and sold plots of land, which were laid out in grid formation, by auction.

THE OPEN PRAIRIE

Pioneers who reminisced about the early days described the land as being treeless except for groves planted to serve as windbreaks for the widely separated farms. One of the pioneers in the region, William George, remembered driving past the Wabasso townsite in 1896: "For miles around these were the only trees to be seen, the rest being all prairie." Cattle were herded from spring through autumn because there were no fences. Joseph Hagert described how he herded cattle as a child. "Both girls and boys had to help with this work," he said. "Each had their own separate herd but all were near together." Still another pioneer, Amandus Georgius, recalled that he herded cattle as a boy because "the land surrounding the farm within a radius of three miles was all prairie." He traveled with his family in a wagon "because it was the best method of conveyance they had. They did not get a buggy until about 1902."

VAIL TOWNSHIP

By the time Wabasso came into being in 1900, my mother's family had already been living for almost three decades on the Daub farm, located in Vail Township approximately two miles north of where the railroad company would found the village. Vail Township was a grassy plain in the center of Redwood County, sparsely populated and undeveloped.

Vail Township had first been named Center Township because it was located in the exact center of the county. Another township had already been named Center, however, so the name was changed to Vail Township, chosen in honor of Fred Vail Hotchkiss, a Redwood Falls blacksmith who was chairman of the Board of Commissioners. The citizens of Vail Township held their first meeting in 1879. At that meeting my maternal grandfather's brother, Theodore Daub, was elected one of two justices for the county. In its first census, carried out in 1880, the population of the township was recorded as 61. By 1890, the population of the township had grown to 213, but there was still no village or town within Vail Township (Table 3).

PRAIRIE FIRE

Frank Johanneck told of a prairie fire that happened in 1891: "At that time Wabasso was unthought of and the country was practically all prairie. There was no railroad and the country was just becoming settled. Prairie fires were quite frequent, usually coming in the fall of the year when all the grass had died off and dried. It was about four o'clock in the afternoon that John Johanneck saw smoke appearing from the south, and at eight o'clock the fire had reached the farm. They had prepared for such an emergency—plowed up a rod of ground around the place, left a portion of the prairie which they burned, and then plowed up another strip a rod wide. This fully protected the place from the prairie fire. At this time Daub's Lake was completely dry and reeds had grown to a height of from twelve to twenty feet. When the fire reached the lake, the flames leaped to a height of at least one hundred feet and the heat could be felt at the Johanneck farm, which is at least a mile from the lake. The flames emitted such a bright light that no lamp was needed in the house. Fire fighting parties were organized among the farmers then living in the country. Crews were formed and already waiting for it. Many haystacks burned but no buildings."

HUNTING

Hunting was popular in the area, not only with the local hunters, who regarded the game as food for their families, but also with sportsmen who came from some distance away. "In the early days, before 1900," said my Uncle Louie Daub, "hunters came by train from Chicago and New York to North Redwood Falls, where they hired triple-seated buggies and drivers to take them hunting. They filled the buggies with prairie chickens, and when the buggies were full, they even had the birds hanging off the sides. They hunted with dogs that they brought with them." Uncle Robert Daub added, "In the fields they made little hummocks of hay over each bird, and at the end of the day they picked up the birds to take back to the hotels in Redwood Falls. They stored their game in refrigerated cars on the trains that took them back east. After the prairie chicken population tapered off, they mostly hunted ducks. The duck and prairie chicken seasons were open at the same time. Daub's Lake and Barnum's Slough were good places for duck hunting. It was a hunter's paradise, with the limit at that time being twenty ducks."

Naming the Village of Wabasso

Wabasso is a Chippewa (Ojibway) word meaning "rabbit" or, perhaps, "white rabbit." The chief engineer for the Western Land Company, which was owned by the Chicago and North Western Railroad Company, named the four small prairie towns that were strung along the railroad line, Wanda, Wabasso, Okawa, and Vesta. The first three names were Chippewa words, chosen in honor of Henry Wadsworth Longfellow's famous poem, *Hiawatha*. The poem about the Chippewa warrior was evidently a favorite of the engineer, and for this reason he chose Chippewa Indian names even though it was the Sioux who were prevalent in the area. The name Okawa was later changed to Seaforth. Vesta, a girl's name, was also the name of the neighboring township in which the village of Vesta was located

.

Platting the Village of Wabasso

The plat for Wabasso was surveyed in 1899, lots were auctioned, and building began immediately. The plat consisted of four whole blocks and two fractions of blocks. The north and south streets, beginning from the west, were named Front, Elm, Oak, Cedar, and Pine. The east and west streets, beginning from the north, were named North, Main, and South. (In the years I lived in Wabasso I cannot remember names for streets other than Main Street being used by anyone, and mail was addressed by neither street name nor house number.) Among the first buildings to go up were the grain elevator and a lumber yard. Stores and businesses, among them a hotel, a livery stable, three blacksmith shops, Dr. H. E. Lucas' drug store, the Bank of Wabasso (the building later became my father's office), and the Liestikow General Store, were established. The town of Wabasso was incorporated in 1900, with a population of 178 persons. The post office was opened, and the *Wabasso Standard*, which has the impressive record of continuing to publish a weekly newspaper ever since its beginning, produced its first issue that same year. Wabasso grew to a population of 343 in 1910; and the population of Vail Township that year was 553.

Because of its central location, Wabasso vied with Redwood Falls for many years in an effort to become the county seat, citing its central location as the reason to move the Redwood County courthouse to Wabasso. Redwood Falls had the advantage of being situated on a water-way. It had been incorporated as a village in 1876, and the railroad arrived in 1878. By 1900, Redwood Falls' population was close to 1000, a number that Wabasso never reached. Redwood Falls pointed out that such a move would cost a great deal of money. A committee of Wabasso citizens got together a petition, and the matter was finally settled in 1919. Wabasso lost the vote by only a very narrow margin, and Redwood Falls remained the county seat.

BACHELOR QUARTERS

"At first," my Uncle Robert Daub told me, "your dad roomed and boarded above the Goblirsch General Store, and he had a little office up there. It was a regular rabbit warren of rooms, and Mrs. Goblirsch had a number of roomers, single men who worked in town and students at the high school. She was a motherly woman who had a big heart. She cooked for them and charged very little. Dr. C. L. Lynn, the first dentist in Wabasso, lived above Goblirsch's store, too. Your father moved out to his office building a few years later, after it became apparent that the practice was going to work out."

Dr. Brey next lived in the Commercial Hotel, which was run by Swan J. Bjorkman, his wife, and their daughters Edla and Hattie. Another daughter Irene, who was married and lived elsewhere, spent a good deal of time with her family and was often present at the Commercial Hotel, too. All of the Bjorkmans were extremely personable and most gracious, so that in later years we children loved to visit "the hotel girls" and their parents. Only my mother restrained her enthusiasm for "the girls"; she seemed to be suspicious that they were a bit too friendly toward my father.

A number of other young bachelors also lived in the Commercial Hotel, among them Dr. Lynn, the dentist, and George Snyder, manager of the lumber yard. Henry Goblirsch, who was courting my mother's sister Clara and who later became my uncle by marriage, was one of the group of friends although he did not live with the others. These young men without immediate families formed a congenial group who tended to look out for one another. This must have been especially helpful to my father, who often made house calls at irregular hours, sometimes when it was sleeting or snowing.

Uncle Louie Daub reported the following incident: "One time your father rode horseback to the Baune farm, five miles out of town, to deliver a baby during a severe winter snowstorm. He turned his horse loose, and the horse came back to town without him. Henry Goblirsch hired a horse and came looking for him. In the meantime, Baune hitched up a team and brought Dr. Brey back to Wabasso. The phone was out of order, or perhaps they didn't have a phone—not many farmers had phones in those days—and there was a lot of confusion before it was all sorted out."

TRANSPORTATION

In the early twentieth century the practice of medicine was undergoing rapid changes, and the emerging automobile was one of the technologies that facilitated these changes. The first successful American gasoline-powered horseless carriage was produced in 1893, and the first mass-produced automobile was manufactured in 1901 by Olds, and around that time a series of articles appeared in the *Journal of the American Medical Association*. Henry Ford marketed the Model C, which he called the official American Doctor's Model, in 1905. The first automobiles not only exposed their occupants to the weather, but they were expensive, difficult to maintain, and far from safe. Poor road conditions were even more of a deterrent to their use. Only a few roads were surfaced, according to the first census of American roads, in 1904, and there were essentially no paved rural roads before 1909. Automobiles were not practical for professional transportation until the Model T appeared on the market in 1908. By 1910 country doctors were turning from their traditional horse and buggy transportation to the automobile.

My father drove a horse and buggy at first, but they were eventually turned over to my mother's father when they were no longer needed. My grandfather Daub never did learn to drive a car, and he was still using the horse (named Bird) and buggy long after everyone else had taken to automobiling. I went with him for a buggy ride only once, when I was about five years old. Covering the distance of two miles from my grandfather's farm to town by open buggy was an exciting adventure, but I most remember the biting wind and bitter cold.

Later my father drove an automobile, his first car being a Model T. "In those days," Uncle Louie told me, "we got around, and this included your dad, mostly by walking. In 1910 there were no county roads, but in 1911 county roads were made with an elevated grader that went back and forth, elevating the roads. Even after that there were very few roads, and those that existed were so muddy that it was impossible to use a car. You can't imagine how terribly muddy the roads were, so bad that most people blocked up their cars and didn't use them during the winter and spring. On many occasions the Daub family walked to town to attend church. I remember one time when my sister, your Aunt Anne, was sick and Dr. Brey walked out to the farm, a distance of two miles, to see her. I took him back to town by horse and buggy after the house call was completed.

"When it was wet, cars were often left at the main road, and people would walk to the farm yards. Sometimes people drove their cars right across the fields or used the meadows to park in. There were lots of meadows and only a few fenced areas for cattle. Of course, when the ground was frozen, one could drive right across the meadows.

"Your dad often had to stop at neighboring farms to ask for directions. I recall an incident when Dr. Brey had parked his car in a meadow late at night. When he returned, he couldn't find his car. The night was pitch-black and also very cloudy. He walked around until daylight, when he was able to locate his car. Another time his car became stuck in the mud. A nearby farmer wearing hip boots pulled him out with a team of horses, but the farmer insisted on being paid in full before he pulled him out."

Uncle Robert contributed a similar anecdote. "After your dad died, your mother asked a certain farmer to settle his bill, which had been incurred about 20 years earlier, $35 for the delivery of a baby. The farmer refused to pay, saying that he had pulled Dr. Brey's car out of the mud or snow, and $35 would just about compensate him for his effort."

Arnold Gadow, a long-time resident of Wabasso, offered further information about how the local physician got around in bad weather. He wrote the following in a Letter to the Editor of the *Wabasso Standard* and in a follow-up letter to me:

> *My father came to Wabasso as foreman on the Chicago and Northwestern railroad. The old section house, an old red house where I spent my entire life, was given to us to use by the railroad.*
>
> *There wasn't hardly any passable roads in those days. I remember how Dr. Brey would come to our house late at night or at 1 or 2 o'clock in the morning and knock on our door. He walked from town, which was about a half mile. I still remember when he came with his long sheep skin coat and fur cap and long warm gloves. He and my father would get the hand car out of the tool shed. It had to be lifted onto the track and my father would start it. It was powered by a gas engine. My father and the doctor would set out in the cold, sometimes 20 degrees or so below zero, many times in stormy weather. Then both would walk side by side to the farm*

place, to see a patient in distress that had to be treated or deliver a baby because Dr. Brey's Model T could not make the trip.

He drove a Model T Ford that had a top that could be taken up and down and it had side flaps to use when needed in all kinds of weather. It was often said that your father would get out of the car and lift it over when he was stuck in mud. He was a powerful man. He was big and also tall.

Arnold Gadow mentioned the sheepskin coat my father wore for protection against the freezing Minnesota weather in winter. My father also had a coat and a pair of mittens made from buffalo hide that he wore only in the very coldest weather, along with a beaver fur hat with ear flaps, when driving an open sled or automobile over snow-covered roads. The buffalo coat is still in the attic of my family home.

THE OFFICE

The office was a small white-painted building located on the south side of Main Street, east of the Commercial Hotel. The building had previously housed a commercial bank. The doctor did not have a nurse or receptionist in the beginning, but he and the dentist assisted each other when necessary. Dr. Brey placed a "business card" in the *Wabasso Standard* at a cost of 75 cents each month. In 1920 a bill from Olaf H. Olson, publisher of the *Wabasso Standard*, Printers, Stationers, Binders, totaled $4.50 for six months.

CITY DRUG STORE

Because small towns commonly had neither a pharmacy nor a pharmacist, it was usual practice for the local physician to both write and fill prescriptions. In preparation for this function, my father had taken not only two pharmacology courses in medical school, but also a pharmacy course entitled "practical pharmacy." The first drug store in Wabasso was conducted by Dr. Herman E. Lucas, the first doctor to locate in Wabasso. Dr. Lucas established a medical practice in 1900 but gave up his practice to run the drug store.

In 1919, with Dr. Lucas' drug store no longer in operation, Dr. Brey bought a building on Main Street across from his office, named it the City Drug Store, and hired Bertha Schottenbauer as manager of the store. At first he filled prescriptions himself. After he sold the City Drug Store to Miss Schottenbauer in 1926, he continued to fill prescriptions for a time, but later a series of pharmacists were hired to work in the drug store.

POLIOMYELITIS

Death rates from poliomyelitis varied from year to year, but there were no major epidemics during the three decades that Dr. Brey practiced medicine in Wabasso. One of his first patients was Pearl Fixsen, the wife of my cousin, John Fixsen. Pearl's daughter, Beatrice Fixsen Emmerick, related the following about her mother's illness, which had always remained vivid in her mind:

"The first time I met your dad was when my mother became sick with polio. It was in the fall of 1910. I was five years old, and my mother was 27. It was during harvest time, and my mother was stacking grain.

"All of a sudden she said, 'Something bit me!' She had felt a sharp pain. She thought nothing of it, but she didn't feel very well for a day or so after that. She was feeling really sort of sick.

"So my father said, 'You'd better hitch up the horse, Old Bess, and go to see the doctor.'

"So she and I went downtown to Wabasso in the horse and buggy to see the doctor. There were two doctors at that time, Dr. Bickford and a new young doctor, whom we didn't know, but he was Frank Brey. (When I was born, on December 9, 1904, there was no doctor, so a midwife took care of the birth.) Well, it happened that Dr. Bickford was out of town, so my mother went to Frank Brey.

"He examined her and said, 'Well, as far as I can see, it appears to be *la grippe*, which is what the flu was called at that time.

"My mother did not get better, so Dr. Bickford, being her own personal doctor, came out to see her when he got back. He said, 'I hate to say this, but I'm afraid you have infantile paralysis.' That's what they called poliomyelitis at that time.

"Now, that was my very first knowledge of Dr. Brey. I remember sitting there in the office on a chair while he had my mother on the table, examining her. Not only did he look at her throat, but he also examined her abdomen, I presume because of her nausea. My mother was in bed for one whole year with the paralysis, and at the end of that time I was six years old."

Poliomyelitis, or infantile paralysis, often begins with mild symptoms similar to those of the common cold or influenza. Fever, sore throat, headache, loss of appetite, nausea, vomiting, and abdominal pain last from a few hours to several days. Cousin Pearl must have been in this early, prodromal phase, when she was first seen. Unfortunately, she had permanent neurological effects that caused her to need a wheelchair for the rest of her days. Signs relating to the nervous system, such as stiff neck and muscle weakness, appear two to six days later, but often do not appear at all. A person who has the early symptoms but never develops neurological signs is said to have a subclinical case, which usually goes undiagnosed. For every person who develops the full-blown disease, it is estimated that between 100 and 800 cases of inapparent disease occur. In the days before poliomyelitis vaccine was available for prevention, subclinical cases accounted for immunity in a substantial portion of the population.

TUBERCULOSIS

Another early patient was my mother's brother, Uncle Louie Daub. He told me about it, as follows: "I contracted tuberculosis of the bowel from the Egle family in 1912 when I was about thirteen years old. I was working at Aunt Lizzie Egle's place because all of the other members of her family had tuberculosis and were too sick to work. That's how I contracted it. Dr. Brey made the diagnosis. First, he gave me a physic of epsom salts—they used a lot of epsom salts in those days—and this seemed to flush everything out. He sent in specimens, but I don't know where they went. Dr. Brey instructed my mother to isolate me from everyone else at home (I slept in the front parlor and the others stayed away), use careful hand washing, launder my linens and clothing in boiling water separately from the family laundry, and dispose of my feces and other body wastes by burying them at a distance from the house. As a result, no one else in my family got tuberculosis."

Two things stand out in Uncle Louie's account. First, no one else in the Daub family contracted tuberculosis, evidently because my Grandmother Daub followed isolation instructions carefully. Second, the story clearly illustrates the reason why my own family never had anything to do with the Egle family. Even though my parents never said a single word against them or their religion, I had always believed it was because the Egles were Protestants. (My Great-aunt Lizzie married a man who was Protestant and joined his church, while my own grandparents, who were both Catholic, remained members of the Church of Rome.) The Egle family was riddled with tuberculosis, and the various members were constantly reported being in and out of tuberculosis sanitariums. My father did not want his wife and children anywhere near any of them.

TABLE 4. *Minnesota population, total deaths from all causes, and death rates per 100,000 population from heart disease and selected communicable diseases 1910-1940. (Chesley AJ and Brower JW, Division of Vital Statistics, Minnesota Department of Health: Live births and rates, deaths and rates, and stillbirths, Minnesota, 1910-1947. Obtained from the Minnesota State Society.)*

Year	Heart Disease	Tuber- culosis	Diph- theria	Polio- myelitis	Typhoid Fever	Deaths All Causes	Minnesota Population
1910	93.2	109.4	27.3	9.7	33.1	22,868	2,075,708
1915	112.8	102.2	9.0	1.2	7.0	22,755	2,231,416
1920	125.0	90.4	10.2	0.8	3.0	25,729	2,387,125
1925	154.5	64.3	9.4	5.9	1.8	25,401	2,475,539
1930	184.1	48.7	1.2	1.4	1.0	25,678	2,563,953
1935	217.8	34.9	0.6	0.4	0.6	26,249	2,678,127
1940	275.5	27.3	0.2	0.9	0.2	26,888	2,792,300

Between 1910 and 1940, tuberculosis was far ahead of all other infectious diseases as a cause of death in Minnesota, with diphtheria running second except in 1910, 1912, and 1913, years when typhoid fever outranked diphtheria (Table 4). There had been a great influx of consumptives into Minnesota after 1850 because the pure, cold air of Minnesota was thought to be salubrious. Large numbers of new settlers came to take advantage of the healthy climate, especially after Henry David Thoreau, who had spent time in Minnesota in 1861 for his consumption, had described the Minnesota River in glowing terms. Some patients had long periods of remission or healed spontaneously, but many died and tuberculosis remained prevalent everywhere. After 1880, as the railroads extended farther west, people who were seeking a healthy climate were more likely to travel to the southwestern states. Minnesota became essentially cleared of tuberculosis during the early 1900s, largely because of strict public health policies that included commitment of infectious patient to sanitariums.

DIPHTHERIA ANTITOXIN

Diphtheria, one of the major causes of death, had been an epidemic disease in earlier centuries, but by the nineteenth and early twentieth centuries it had become endemic in cities. Diphtheria was greatly feared; and when the antitoxin became available, it represented an important medical advance. The bacterium responsible for causing diphtheria was identified in 1884 by Klebs and Loeffler, and in 1889 Yersin and Roux showed that the damage from diphtheria is caused chiefly by toxins produced by the bacteria. This was the first bacterial disease for which a toxic cause was identified. In 1890 Behring developed an antitoxin that effectively neutralized the toxin, so that the antitoxin could be used clinically to treat patients who had the disease and to give immediate immunity to persons who had been exposed to the disease. Thus, diphtheria was the first bacterial disease for which a vaccine was used for treatment and short-term prevention. Several decades later, diphtheria became the first infectious disease against which a toxoid vaccine was used successfully to give long-term immunity.

Dr. Brey, as the Health Officer in Wabasso, was in charge of a distribution station for free diphtheria antitoxin, which was supplied by the Minnesota State Board of Health. He was obligated to account for every vial of vaccine that was used. He recorded the amounts of vaccine received and made out an individual form for each patient to whom vaccine was administered. Doses of 1,000 units were considered to be prophylactic (preventive) doses, for persons who had been exposed to diphtheria. Doses of 5,000 units or more were considered to be therapeutic (treatment) doses, for persons who had clinical evidence of diphtheria. Outdated material was returned to the Board of Health. Among his papers were an undated instruction sheet from the Minnesota State Board of Health [Figure 20 a,b], his inventory reports for 1920, 1921, 1922, and 1924 (Table 5), and sheaves of report forms for patients for the years 1917 through 1925.

On one occasion he received, rather than administered, a dose of diphtheria antitoxin. On July 30, 1917, he filled out a form for himself,

TABLE 5. *Inventory of free diphtheria antitoxin vials (Lederle brand) on hand in Dr. Brey's station at various times. Receipts were required for each vial that was used, and outdated material was returned to the Minnesota Board of Health.*

Date	1,000 Units	5,000 Units	10,000 Units
October 15, 1920	8	6	0
September 6, 1921	8	6	0
November 25, 1922	8	5	0
January 6, 1924	13	18	26

a 31-year-old male, for a prophylactic (preventive) dose of 1000 units. He had no doubt been exposed to a patient with the full-blown disease, perhaps little seven-year-old Elnora W., who had been given a therapeutic (treatment) dose of 5000 units on July 2. Administration of the antitoxin, obtained from horse serum, can be hazardous. If a patient has been sensitized to horse serum, most probably through previous exposure to horse serum, he or she could have an allergic reaction. The most severe reaction that could occur would be anaphylactic shock, causing the blood pressure to plummet suddenly and rapidly, resulting in death unless epinephrine (adrenaline) is administered immediately. He might not have appreciated the danger of a possible reaction.

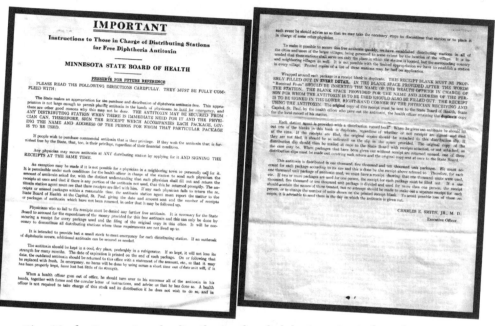

Fig. 20a,b: *Instructions for distributing free diphtheria antitoxin from the Minnesota State Board of Health. The date was August 11, 1920.*

In the early days before he had an office nurse, he carried out all procedures himself. He and the town's only dentist were accustomed to assisting each other; for example, he often administered the anesthetic if Dr. Lynn had a patient with a difficult dental problem. One would hope that when he gave himself a dose of diphtheria antitoxin, Dr. Lynn was standing by with epinephrine in a syringe, in case a reaction occurred. At any rate, there is no evidence that Dr. Brey ever again, in spite of the repeated exposures he must have had, received diphtheria antitoxin.

Frequently the antitoxin was administered to whole families, with larger doses being given to the patients who were ill and smaller doses to the family members who had been exposed. A youth who appeared to be active and somewhat unwilling was 12-year-old Louie E., who was first given a therapeutic dose of diphtheria antitoxin in 1920. During the procedure, a 5,000 unit vial was "broken, in attempting to administer." Young Louie, by now 15 years of age, came to attention again in 1923. A vial, this one containing 1,000 units of the antitoxin, was again "lost, broken while administering." That young man must have been a handful!

RECREATION

Dr. Brey's favorite pastimes took place out of doors and his frequent hunting and fishing companions were my mother's brothers and Dr. Lynn, as well as Father Francis Roemer, the pastor of St. Anne's Catholic Church in Wabasso. He had a set of six duck decoys, two drakes and four ducks; each of us children inherited one. My two brothers have the drakes, and my three sisters and I have the ducks. Mention of his hunting and fishing companions brings up an interesting sidelight. Although in my memory my father attended church only once a year, on Easter Sunday, one of his dearest friends was the local Catholic priest, Father Roemer.

"Your dad hunted ducks on Daub's Lake and Barnum's Slough, which was an especially good slough for ducks," said Uncle Louie Daub. "By this time the land was plowed over, and the prairie chickens had disappeared. His dog was a white hunting dog with black spots named Sport. Later, in 1924, he had a police dog, also called a German shepherd, named Queenie. He didn't go deer hunting. Doc, John (Daub, my brother), and I fished together on Lake Sarah. On one occasion Dr. Brey and Father Roemer brought a bunch of bullheads and pickerel home and put them in the (water) tank at Daub's farm. We had fresh fish for awhile."

Uncle Robert added, "We fished in Daub's Lake with a net. This was not really legal but it was commonly done. I remember one time, when I was about nine years old, going fishing with your dad and Dr. Lynn. They used dynamite to stun the fish, and on one occasion your dad became very sick from whiffs of the dynamite fumes. This was before he was married, and Dr. Lynn called in Elizabeth to care for him."

TEMPER, TEMPER

My father usually tried to keep his temper tamped down, but he was not always successful, as illustrated by an anecdote told by an elderly resident of the Wabasso Health Care Center, the nursing home in Wabasso. Dr. Brey frequently became irritated with Nick Franta, one of the local business men, she said, and, on one occasion after a disagreement, he called Mr. Franta a "son of a bitch." Nick retaliated by taking him to court, where the judge slapped a ten-dollar fine upon my father "for calling a citizen an unwarranted name."

"Is it all right to think he's a son of a bitch?" inquired young Dr. Brey of the judge.

"You may think anything you like," replied the judge, "but you may not say anything you like."

"It was worth every cent it cost," declared my father, "to call the son of a bitch a son of a bitch!"

A similar anecdote was related to me with a chuckle by Father Michael Guetter, who was then living in Wabasso as a retired Catholic priest. (Father Guetter noted parenthetically that he had been delivered by my father in 1915.) Nick Franta and another man were sitting on a bench in front of Dr. Brey's office, making disparaging remarks about the doctor. Unknown to them, he heard what they were saying. The doctor filled a pail with cold water, carried it outside, dumped it over the head of the surprised Mr. Franta, and returned to his office, all of this without speaking a word. In another version of this story that I heard later, Nick was complaining about the hot weather while sitting under a shade tree on the side of the street on which the office was located. The incident happened around 1934, a number of years after the court appearance. No one has ever been able to tell me how the enmity between the men began. One thing is sure, however: the townfolk must have had a wonderful time passing these stories around.

EDUCATION

Throughout his lifetime, my father was concerned with education, and in his early bachelor years he gave a great deal of encouragement to members of his own family. He tried to interest his young relatives in going on to school beyond their high school years, often offering to lend them money for expenses. Arlean Schwing, his first cousin, wrote about her sister Susie:

"In our family, Susie was the one who was the closest to him because she used to go to Wabasso to visit relatives and that gave her a chance to visit with him. Susie used to tell me that your dad wanted Susie to take up nursing. She told him she couldn't do that because she didn't have the money. Your dad said he would loan her the money, but she said she was afraid of having a loan, and then something might develop so she couldn't pay it off. Susie was very afraid that way. We were always told, 'if you haven't got the money, don't go into debt.'"

Dr. Brey had better success with other young relatives. With help and encouragement from his Uncle Frank, my cousin Irving Brey, Uncle Louie Brey's son, completed his education at Creighton University in Nebraska and qualified as a pharmacist. In later years, several grand nephews not only finished college but went on to earn advanced degrees.

THE DOCTOR AS PATIENT

My father was an exceptionally strong and healthy person, and I never knew him to be sick before his final illness. He had been hospitalized once, however, prior to his marriage, in Worrell Hospital, in Rochester. His Mayo Clinic record (# 0-358-859) described him as a 35-year-old, single male (he married later that year). Listed as his closest relative was his "father, 6th St. N. Broadway, New Ulm." He was charged $6.00 per day for 4¾ days to a total of $29.00, and a $6.00 operating room fee was added to make a final total of $35.00 [Figure 21].

He had been examined on Monday, May 23, 1921, by Dr. Rockwell, otolaryngology consultant, who noted :

"Chief Complaint: Repeated sore throats. Many years duration. Chronic nasal obstruction, less severe in summer. No nasal discharge. Nose feels dry. Sense of smell diminished. Trouble present over many years. General health good. No other complaints. Influenza 2½ years ago [this is the only indication I have ever been aware of that he had been ill with the flu in 1918]. Not seriously ill at that time.

"Summary: Septic tonsils and chronic hypertrophic rhinitis. Thickened deviated septum a factor in nasal condition.

"Advise: General examination. Tonsils. Submucous resection [there is no evidence that a submucous resection was ever carried out]."

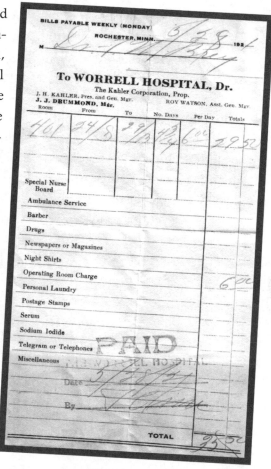

Fig. 21: *Bill from Worrell Hospital, Rochester, Minnesota, for Dr. Brey's hospitalization from May 24 to 29, 1921.*

He was examined on the same day by Dr. D. M. Berkman, physician, who noted the following:

"Clinical history: Negative general history. To be OK'd for tonsillectomy.

"Examination: Negative. SBP (systolic blood pressure) 120; DBP (diastolic blood pressure) 70; pulse 66. OK for tonsillectomy."

His tonsillectomy took place on April 25, 1921, and the operating surgeon, Dr. Lyons, noted the following:

"Septic tonsils. Tonsillectomy. Very large, fibrous, septic tonsils, removed with the Robertson knife and snare. Two ligatures each fossa."

Along with the hospital bill, he saved the Mayo Clinic operating room schedules for Tuesday, May 24 [Figure 22] (his procedure was carried out the following day) and Friday, May 27 [Figure 23], as well as a follow-up letter from Dr. Monte Piper. (Dr. Piper's letter concerned an invitation to hunt in the Wabasso area and offered concrete evidence that the prairie chickens had not yet deserted southern Minnesota.) The Mayo operating rooms were clearly set up for observation, and visiting physicians were welcomed. The schedules informed visitors: "The first row of seats is reserved for members of the staff and doctors wearing gowns."

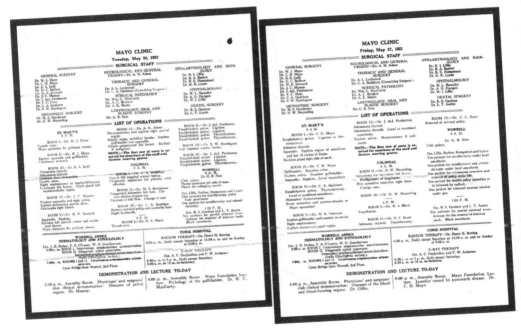

(From Left To Right)
Fig. 22: *Mayo Clinic operating schedule for Tuesday, May 24, 1921. Dr. William J. Mayo was operating that day.*

Fig. 23: *Mayo Clinic operating schedule for Friday, May 27, 1921. Dr. Charles H. Mayo was operating that day.*

CONTINUING MEDICAL EDUCATION (CME)

Long before continuing medical education (CME) was required by state medical licensing boards, the Mayo Clinic was offering interested physicians the opportunity to learn about new medical and surgical treatments. Dr. Brey obviously took advantage of the Clinic's willingness to teach, and observing tonsillectomies may have given him the impetus to begin performing the procedure in his own office. One of his penciled notes on the back of the May 27 schedule reminds himself to purchase: lamp bulb 150 wat [sic] 110 volt, scopolamin [sic], tonsil haemostat [sic], and light bulbs 150 volts, as well as white ointment and hankerchiefs [sic]. It mentions the use of thyroxin to treat the myxoedema [sic] type of goiter. Another penciled note lists the supplies and methods that would be needed for tonsillectomies performed under local anesthesia: 1/200 scopolamin [sic], 1/8 morphin [sic] one-half hour before local anesthetic cocaine 1/5 of 1% with 1 drop of adrenalin in 1 dram or 60 drops—boil the cocaine but not adrenalin—can inject 2 to 4 drams.

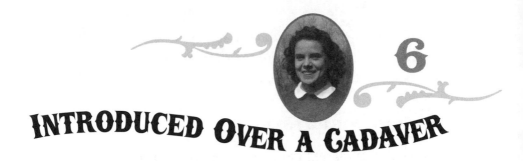

INTRODUCED OVER A CADAVER

Fran and I are the only couple I know who met over a cadaver. We owe this to our classmate Ethel Erickson. She was from northern Minnesota, of Finnish descent, very blond, and older than most of the students in the class. Trained as a medical technician, Ethel had worked in New York for a number of years before applying to medical school. After graduation from medical school, she became a forensic pathologist and performed autopsies on some famous people, including Howard Hughes. "Eric" was a motherly sort of person; she had met Fran earlier, and she decided that he and I should get to know each other. We worked in groups of four in gross anatomy laboratory, dissecting our cadavers. One day she took Fran by the hand, brought him to the room in gross anatomy lab in which three of my classmates and I were dissecting our cadaver, and formally introduced us in front of everyone in the room.

FIRST DATE

Our romance didn't get off to a smooth start. Fran cancelled our first date, saying that he had to go to his grandmother's funeral. I learned later that he really did go to his grandmother's funeral. We eventually had our first date, which consisted of a Chinese dinner and a movie downtown. I was impressed that we went and came home by taxicab. In those days students were not allowed to have cars on the University of Minnesota campus, and we were accustomed to going places by street car. A taxicab ride was a special treat.

FRATERNITY BROTHERS

Fran lived at the Phi Chi house, a beautiful brick building across the street from the medical school; the building is still there. I was occasionally invited to parties at the house, learned to play bridge there, and eventually came to know most of his fraternity brothers quite well. Tony Ourada, Andy Midthune, Bob Clark, Winston Lindberg, Bob Rocknem, Lyle Jacobson, Jennings Peteler, and Raymond Read were fun to be with and, I'm sure, knowing them protected me from the displeasure of other students who resented women being in the class.

One of Fran's fraternity brothers, who later became famous as the first surgeon to perform open heart surgery, was C. Walton Lillehei. Walt was unmarried and older than most of the students who lived in the house. He had finished medical school, completed his military service, and was serving a surgery residency under the chairman of surgery, Dr. Owen H. Wangensteen. Two other important and well known faculty members Walt worked with in the Department of Surgery at that time were Richard Varco and Clarence Dennis. Walt was dating Kaye. She was a slender, young, attractive, graduate nurse, as all airline stewardesses for Northwest Airlines were required to be. About that time Northwest Airlines instituted an additional policy of requiring flight attendants to be unmarried, but those who were already married could stay on if they married before the January 1st deadline of the coming year. Kaye and Walt were married one New Year's Eve, to avoid the deadline, and Walt moved out of the fraternity house.

A MISSED DIAGNOSIS

Walt was always very pleasant to me, as he was to everyone, but I had only known him socially. When I encountered him during my surgery clerkship as a junior in medical school, I found out how professional Dr. Lillehei could be! He assigned me to take a medical history and perform a physical examination on a woman of late middle age. This was my first experience dealing with a patient, and I was very nervous. I really couldn't find anything wrong with her, but when I reported that she had had a recent weight loss of ten pounds, he pounced on her history. Ten pound weight loss! He carefully examined the woman and found a large mass in her abdomen that I had missed. I was so embarrassed that I wanted to sink through the floor. He operated on her and removed a large cancer of the stomach. After that he gave me an updated report concerning the patient every time I met him in the hallways. He always spoke in a most kindly and friendly manner, and I should have welcomed the information, but all I wanted was to hear no more about my mistake!

A WEDDING

Fran and I dated through medical school, became engaged in 1945, and were married in the chapel of the University of Minnesota on September 21, 1946. I received my Bachelor of Medicine degree three months later, in December, 1946. At that time the University of Minnesota conferred the Doctor of Medicine degree after an internship was completed. Thus, Fran, who had received his MB degree in March, 1946, received his MD degree in December, 1946, at the same time I received my MB degree.

IN-LAWS

Fran disappointed his parents, Thomas and Frances Haddy, who were immigrants from Lebanon, because they had hoped their new daughter-in-law would be a girl of Lebanese descent. His older brother, Joe, had already disappointed them by marrying a non-Lebanese girl. However, Fran's mother and father, along with his sister Beatrice and cousin DeLayne Shaheen, attended our wedding and were gracious to everyone in my family. DeLayne was Fran's best man.

Fran's parents, who were Christian, had left Lebanon because of religious persecution. They came from a small Christian Orthodox town called Ain Arab, one of many small towns scattered throughout their area. The people in the various towns segregated themselves by religion, whether Christian, Muslim, or Druse. The Druse (or Druze) religion, which is somewhat mysterious, is a religious sect originating among Muslims and centered in the mountains of Lebanon and Syria. While Fran's dad worked as a boy tending sheep on the mountainside, young Druse men carrying guns would customarily harass him from horseback. The final impetus to emigrate came because he was scheduled to be inducted into the Turkish Army. The military was a dangerous place to be. It was not unusual for young Christian men to be killed, not by the enemy, but by persons on their own side. With his parents' permission, he left Lebanon alone at 17 years of age and headed for the United States. He first met Fran's mother as a young girl who was emigrating with her parents on the same ship. They met again and married when they were older. Fran's father became a successful businessman in Kiester, Minnesota, eventually owning a general merchandise store there and two more in little towns near Kiester.

There is an interesting story about how Fran got his name. He was the fifth child born to his parents. Elizabeth, Beatrice, Lucille, and Joe were older, and his twin sisters, Juanita and Vernita, came along later. He was scheduled to be named Thomas, after his father, if he turned out to be a boy. However, his dad was out of town on business when he arrived, and his mother, angry at his father's absence, announced that this baby boy would instead be named Francis (with an "i") after her. Whenever the story was told, Fran remarked, "I wish my father had stayed home!"

BIG RED HOUSE ON THE HILL

In 1946 my mother and siblings bought a big red house on the hill across the street from Langford Park in St. Paul, near the University of Minnesota St. Paul Campus, better known as the "Farm" Campus. My father had always talked about his plan to buy a house adjacent to the U of M so that my five siblings and I could attend the university. He expected all of us to go to college, he said, but he could not afford to send all of us to private colleges. Tuition at the state university would be minimal, and we could save money by living at home. The house was an old Queen Anne Victorian house built in 1895 with three parlors, five bedrooms, an attic, and a basement. We paid $10,000 for the house, which came mostly from selling our house in Wabasso, and which we thought was a lot of money. Three of us, Ann, Paul, and I, received degrees from the University of Minnesota. Al attended the agricultural college for several years before returning to Wabasso to work the farm my mother inherited from my father. Virginia graduated from St. Catherine's College with a degree in nursing. Justine decided not to go to college. A number of cousins and friends of the family lived in the Red House while they attended the U of M. Fran and I lived in the house while he finished his internship and I finished medical school. I lived there as an intern, and later as a pediatric resident with our son, Rick.

UPHOLDING THE LAW

The electrocardiogram was invented by William Einthoven in the Netherlands in 1903. August Wasserman in Germany developed a test for syphilis in 1906, and Paul Ehrlich, also in Germany, discovered salvarsan (arsphenamine, an arsenic compound) treatment for the disease in 1910. Microscopic methods for examining the blood, urine, and sputum were introduced into the University of Minnesota College of Medicine and Surgery in 1900. Digitalis, produced from the purple foxglove plant, had been used for the treatment of congestive heart failure since its introduction by William Withering in England during the late eighteenth century. Amyl nitrate was first used for angina pectoris by Sir Thomas Lauder Bunton, also in England, in the nineteenth century. Better control of heart failure resulted from several improvements in treatment during the early twentieth century: more effective usage of digitalis and its components, including digoxin; more efficient dosage schedules; and the employment of mercurial diuretics. Heparin was discovered at Johns Hopkins University between 1911 and 1916. Moses Barron at the University of Minnesota proved that diseased Islets of Langerhans in the pancreas caused diabetes mellitus.

Dr. Frank W. Brey served as coroner, at first appointed and later elected to the office, for Redwood County from March 12, 1914, through January 4, 1926. As a medical student, his course in pathology included time spent in the "dead house," where he learned under supervision how to perform an autopsy. He also completed a course in medical jurisprudence, which the University of Minnesota Medical School had required of its students from the time it opened in 1888. His medical school training, as well as his access to the resources of the University of Minnesota for chemical tests and pathological tissue evaluations, must have helped him to feel confident that he could carry out the duties of this office.

"CROWNERS"

Originally called "Crowners" because their chief duty was to collect any fines or death duties due the crown, that is, the king, they eventually became known as coroners. Most sources agree that the office of coroner was established in England in 1195, for the purpose of collecting money to liberate King Richard I (1189-1199), who was being held for ransom by Leopold of Austria. Other authors date the office to the even earlier time of King Alfred (871-910). Coroners' duties were mostly legal and administrative. They were obliged to investigate deaths that occurred suddenly or unexpectedly or were suspicious in any way. The coroner was rarely a physician, but he could request that a physician, usually a surgeon, examine a body and perform an autopsy if indicated. The coroner system in colonial America was copied from the English system. The medical and legal aspects gradually became separated, and the office of medical examiner was established. In 1877 Massachusetts became the first state to require a medical degree for its medical examiner.

CORONER'S DUTIES

When a death appeared to be violent or unnatural, or when the cause was unknown, the coroner was obligated to carry out an investigation. The coroner could come to a decision on his own after looking at external, objective evidence and taking statements from witnesses, or an autopsy could be requested if in his judgment it was appropriate. If there was a question between an accident or suicide, or if there was a possibility that a crime had been committed, the coroner was obligated to summon witnesses and assemble jurors for an inquest.

Before 1880, very little attention was given to workmen who were injured or killed on the job. Although railway construction, for example, paid workmen very well, railroad contractors were not held responsible for compensating work-related accidents. As a result of the industrial revolution and increasing urbanization of the early 1880s, the responsibility of employers in the case of accidental deaths began to be emphasized by the middle and late 1880s, and inquests began to focus on occupational accidents.

DR. BREY AS CORONER

The minutes of the Redwood County Board of Commissioners for a special session commencing March 12, 1914, reported Dr. Brey's appointment as coroner: "On motion of H. M. Aune duly passed, the resignation of Dr. F. W. Aldrich as coroner was accepted. The board proceeded to appoint a County Coroner, and Dr. F. W. Brey of Wabasso was duly appointed and so declared by the Chairman. The Bond of the Coroner was fixed at $1,000.00 on motion of H. M. Aune duly passed." The appointment was confirmed at the session commencing January 5, 1915, according to the minutes of that meeting. "The official bond of Frank W. Brey as County Coroner in the amount of $1,000 with George Franta and Dayton E. Billings as sureties was presented, and on motion of John Arends duly passed, bond and sureties were approved." He was elected to the post in 1918 and re-elected in 1922.

Among his papers is a Certificate of Election signed and witnessed with "my hand and Official Seal at Redwood Falls in said County this [blank] day of November A. D. 1922" by S. N. Larson, County Auditor, Redwood County, Minn., that Frank W. Brey, Wabasso, Minn. "received the highest number of votes cast for the office of County Coroner in the County of Redwood and State of Minnesota and was therefore duly elected to said office as appears from the official election returns and canvass, on file in my office." This election had been held just two weeks before his first child, my sister Ann, was born. She was four years old, and two more of us had arrived, when he decided not to run again for office in 1926.

REDWOOD COUNTY RECORDS

Several documents help to fill out the picture of his work as county coroner. Appendix C contains a chronologically numbered list of actions taken from Redwood County court records, but the list is by no means a complete record of the coroner's activities. This appendix is of interest because it demonstrates causes of death in Redwood County for that time period. His billing record, also found among his papers, states that his reimbursement cost per mile was $0.10. For two periods from December, 1916, to May 3, 1919, and from December 23, 1916, to February 20, 1923, his travel reimbursement requests were $366.90 and $662.50.

Not surprisingly, in a relatively sparsely populated area such as Redwood County, serious crimes were uncommon. Reports from two of his earliest cases were retained among his papers, the apparent suicide of Carl Nelson, which was submitted by an acting coroner, and the industrial accident of Edward A. Laudert, in which he himself functioned as coroner. Although autopsies were performed upon occasion, unfortunately, no example of an actual autopsy record has survived. The cases that follow serve as further examples of a coroner's work in rural Minnesota in the early twentieth century.

WHO WAS POISONED WITH STRYCHNINE?

The fatal strychnine poisoning must have been one, perhaps the first, of his important cases. A mysterious letter from J. H. Derby, Department of Chemistry, University of Minnesota, to Dr. F. W. Brey, County Coroner, dated Oct. 23, 1916, states that "Your letter [and]... the contents of an Express package you had shipped for analysis" had been turned over to him by Dean G. B. Frankforter. After performing the analysis in his private laboratory, Dr. Derby reported the presence of strychnine in the enclosed samples of urine and internal organs, including liver, kidney, stomach, spleen, etc., but not in the enclosed sausages. Neither the letter nor the report included the name of a patient. His bill for $150, to be paid to an analytical chemist in St. Paul, was enclosed.

An answer is found in the local newspapers. The September 14, 1916, issue of the *Morgan Messenger* carried the story of William Harder, a retired "pioneer of the community," who had been living alone, mentioning that the coroner and the jury for an inquest awaited information from the "state chemist." The September 20, 1916, issue of the *Redwood Gazette* stated, "William Harder, who died last Sunday evening, was buried Monday afternoon, September 18. The relatives were given permission to bury the deceased although they had not yet heard from the state chemist. The coroner held an inquist [sic] and a jury was picked which has not yet been discharged."

Dr. J. L. Adams of Morgan, Minnesota, sent a notarized bill, dated June 8, 1918, for $15.00 for performing an "Autopsy on the body of William Harder on Sept. 11, 1916." No copy of the autopsy report has been found. Since no further information appeared in any of the newspapers, it seems likely that, following the inquest on December 21, 1916, the death was ruled a suicide.

ALBERT HEIMAN AND CLYDE SLOUGH

On November 6, 1916, two men lost their lives in a railroad accident, one of the worst that had ever happened in Redwood County. At a railroad crossing near Lamberton, the seven o'clock freight train struck a truck carrying a crew of workmen. Albert Heiman and Clyde Slough were killed and several other men were injured. A detailed description of the accident made the front page of the *Redwood Gazette* on November 8th and in the *Lamberton Star* on November 10th.

The coroner immediately directed the following notice "To any Constable of said County from the state of Minnesota, County of Redwood, Greeting: You are hereby commanded immediately to summon six good and lawful men to appear before me, the Coroner of said County at Lamberton, Minn.: Math Miesen, I C Strinkauser, Leo Roth, Wm C Roth, A A Swanbeck, and G A Shunck, on the 6th day of Nov A. D. 1916 at 11 o'clock AM, then and there to inquire, upon view of the body [sic] of Albert Heiman and Clyde Slough there lying dead, how and by what means he [sic] came to his [sic] death; hereof fail not. Given under my hand this 6th day of Nov A. D. 1916, F W Brey, Coroner of Redwood County."

A notice dated the same day was directed by "The People of the State of Minnesota to the Sheriff or any Constable in said County to summon witnesses Harley Gooler and Mrs. Wm York to appear before a Coroner's inquest to be held at Lamberton on the 9th day of Nov A. D. 1916 at 9 o'clock in the forenoon, to testify and the truth to speak in behalf of and concerning the matter of the death of Albert Heiman and Clyde Slough." The inquest actually took place on Dec 21.

THE KLEEMAN FAMILY

One of two high profile crimes that involved the county coroner was a gruesome multiple murder and suicide on a farm near Clements. The *Redwood Gazette* described the tragedy on March 28, 1917. Four days earlier, a young husband and father had killed his wife and four children, ages six weeks through five years, each with a single blow upon the head from an ax, as they lay sleeping, and then hanged himself in the kitchen. The bloody scene was discovered by a school teacher, who roomed and boarded with the family, when she returned from a weekend away.

CHARLES E. LAMBERTON

The other crime that received intense publicity occurred when two rival Redwood Falls businessmen who had a long history of disagreement, William Rosendahl and Charles E. Lamberton, had a dispute on June 24, 1917, which ended in a fight. According to the June 27, 1917, issue of the *Redwood Gazette*, Lamberton died of a gunshot wound from Rosendahl's gun. The fatal shooting was observed by the chief of police, Carl Byram, who had known of their altercation and followed the men. Rosendahl was immediately arrested and subsequently convicted and sentenced to jail.

CARL NELSON

Carl Nelson was evidently a homeless man who hanged himself in a barn that belonged to a Sherman Township farmer named Christ Jensen on November 18, 1918. The report submitted by J. L. Adams, M. D., Acting Coroner indicated that, "Examination of premises and witness preclude any suspicion of foul play or criminal carelessness on the part of anyone." The statements of two witnesses, Christ Jensen and a neighbor, were included. No autopsy was considered necessary. Dr. Adams searched the body, deposited $75.82 found in his clothing in the bank, and authorized undertaker Nels Jensen of Morgan, Minn., to give the body a decent burial in the Village Cemetery at Morgan, Minn. Dr. Adams noted that he forwarded a letter found on the body from Carl Nelson's only living relative, a sister living in Copenhagen, to her along with a notification of his death. The *Morgan Messenger* reported the death as a suicide, making special note of Mr. Nelsen's tendency to melancholy and inclination to brood over his "weakness for King Alcohol." On February 10, 1919, M. R. Merring, Attorney at Law, Morgan, Minn., sent a copy of the investigation of the death to Dr. F. W. Brey, along with a claim from K. M. Jensen, undertaker for a balance of $27.18.

DORIS MAURER

On November 16, 1919, the body of Doris Maurer, with a bullet wound in her head, was found by a visitor. A young foster daughter, unharmed, was present in the same room. It was thought that the death had occurred either the day before or that same day. The woman's husband was out of town with a number of companions on a fishing trip. Because no motive for suicide was known and the possibility of murder was suggested, the following six jurors were immediately summoned "on November 16, 1919, at 10 am, to view the body of Doris Maurer": Oscar Goetze, John Whitcomb, George Lamphere, Kenneth Mackenzie, Edgar Garruth, Wm Smith. The following witnesses were summoned to appear before a Coroner's inquest "on November 20, 1919, at 10:00 am to give evidence in behalf of and concerning the matter of the death of Doris Maurer: Minnie Lamphere, Mrs Thomas (Mary) McCormick, Thomas McCormick, Wm S. Maurer, Dr. W A Conland, and Harry Beaty." The decision of the jury was preempted by the *Redwood Gazette*, which announced the day before the inquest, "Young woman kills herself by shooting late Saturday or early Sunday."

EDWARD A. LAUDERT

On February 23, 1923, Dr. F. W. Brey held an inquest in the Village Hall in the Village of Sanborn on the body of Edward A. Laudert, who died on February 11, 1923, in a railroad accident. The neatly indexed report states that the jury consisted of the following six persons: C. C. Ripley, Wm Woehrman, Fred Manecke, W. J. Becker, H. H. Peake, and Christ Phelan.

Witnesses who were called by the coroner to give their testimony included the following:

Dr. H. M. Joergens, a practicing physician who gave emergency medical care to the injured man.

George Book, engineer in charge of the train.

Claude M. Titus, fireman on the train.

Arno Herman Loose, brakeman on the train.

C. P. Nissen, conductor on the train.

Herman J. Yeager, a witness who lived in Sanborn and was called to help care for the injured man.

John G. Leopold, round-house wiper.

Lloyd L. Barnes, car foreman.

R. H. Wulf, in charge of the hotel to which the injured man was taken.

The report of the inquest occupied 39 typewritten pages. The final verdict, signed by F. W. Brey, Coroner, C. B. Fraser, Deputy Coroner, and all six of the jurors was: "said Edward A. Laudert died from shock and internal injuries caused by being caught and crushed between two box cars on railroad track of the Chicago Northwestern Railway Company in west end of yards at Sanborn, Minnesota, one of said cars being attached to an engine of said company moving eastward on main line and one of said cars standing on side track of said company in said railroad yard, the first car attached to engine having left track of main line." The *Sanborn Sentinel* carried a detailed description of the accidental death on February 15, 1923, stating, "Why one of the cars should have left the track when it did is a mystery."

For his excellent "stenographic report of Inquest over Body of William A. Laudert ($17.10) and Mileage Sanborn & Return to Redwood Falls ($5.00)," Walter W. White submitted a bill for $22.10.

External examination and objective evidence was considered sufficient for this report, and no autopsy was required.

COURT COSTS

It seems quite certain that Dr. Brey was not salaried for his work as coroner, but he evidently expected to be paid a flat fee of $5.00 plus travel reimbursement of $0.10 per mile for each case or instance that required his presence. He seems to have sent statements infrequently. It is not clear whether he received payments in response to the statements.

The costs for coroner's inquests are listed in Redwood County's financial statements. For example, under DISBURSEMENTS, costs were listed as $56.65 in 1915, $15 in 1918, and $82.04 in 1919 for coroner's fees or coroner's inquests.

Although his reimbursement appears to be minimal in terms of the value of today's dollars, it may have been a useful contribution to his income. It can be assumed, however, that Dr. Brey considered his work as coroner to be a community service. He served through 1926, when a new coroner was elected. The minutes of the board dated January 4, 1927, note that a bond was posted for the newly elected coroner, A. U. Hubbard. My father had no doubt decided by then that his busy practice and family life would preclude his continuing as coroner. He may also have wished to be more directly involved with children and their education in his community. Shortly afterward, in 1929, he became a member of the Wabasso School Board, where he continued to serve until his death in 1940.

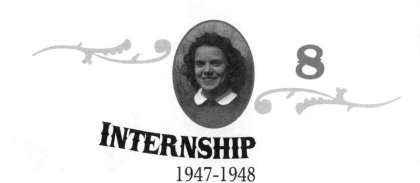

INTERNSHIP
1947-1948

F ran received his MB degree in March, 1946, and started a rotating internship at the Minneapolis General Hospital (MGH) in April. He received his Doctor of Medicine (MD) degree in December, 1946, and I received my Bachelor of Medicine (MB) degree at the same time. During those years the University of Minnesota did not award the Doctor of Medicine (MD) degree until an approved internship was completed. Fran finished his internship on June 30, 1947, and I started mine the next day, July 1 [Figure 24]. I had been accepted for a rotating internship, too, but, I had to wait for six months before I could start. I spent the six months on Dr. A. B. Baker's neurology service at the University of Minnesota Hospitals. Dr. Baker was a dynamic teacher whose teaching was always interesting and stimulating. He was not prejudiced against women, quite the opposite; in fact, his chief resident was a woman, Faye Tichy.

THE MINNEAPOLIS GENERAL HOSPITAL

Everybody loved the MGH. Morale was high, everyone worked hard, and we all learned a lot about medicine and how to deal with patients. The patients, except some who came to the Emergency Room, were mostly indigent or low income. They tended to appreciate the services they received, or were, at any rate, not big complainers. We were paid $15 a month plus room and board. We were fed four times each

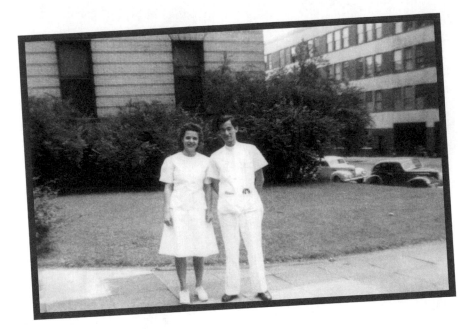

Fig. 24: *Drs. Fran and Terry Haddy in front of the Minneapolis General Hospital, July1, 1947.*

day, with the full dinner served at midnight being our favorite meal. I was assigned a room in the MGH nurses' quarters, but I slept there only when I was on call and went home the other nights.

We were immediately supervised by our chief residents, who were usually in their third year of residency, although on the surgical services we were more likely to report to a fourth or fifth year resident. Our ultimate supervisors were either faculty members at the University of Minnesota Medical School or private physicians who practiced in Minneapolis. They came to make teaching rounds two or three time a week, and most of them did not come in for any other reason. The chief residents I had were exceptionally competent, especially when one considers that most of them were not long past their own internships, and they were all caring, and compassionate. The MGH patients received excellent medical care during the years I was there.

Our working schedule usually consisted of working all day and taking call every third or fourth night, depending upon how many interns were assigned to the particular service we were on. When we were on night call, we often worked most of the night, sometimes all night long, if the service was a busy one. When we were up all night, we were expected to show up for morning rounds at 8:00 am (on the surgical services 7:00 am), looking bright and attentive and ready to start a full day's work. Fran had the experience of rotating as an intern through the busy infectious disease service during the 1946-1947 poliomyelitis epidemic. For his three-day rotation he worked all day and all night the first day, all day and until midnight the second day, and all day until 5:00 pm the third day. For each three-day period, he had 16 hours to sleep and eight hours to carry out personal errands.

Up All Night

Among my patients who kept me up all night long was a middle-aged man who was bleeding from esophageal varicosities. When the liver becomes fibrous from alcoholism, as his did, the blood flow in the liver is obstructed, and the blood vessels leading to and from the liver, located in the lining of the esophagus, become distended and often bleed. The patient, of course, was terrified. He was losing a lot of blood, and the only option was to replace the lost blood with red blood cell transfusions until the bleeding could be stopped. Administering blood transfusions through an arm vein as fast as he was losing it from bleeding was a challenge that kept me running back and forth from the blood bank all night long. He made it through the night, and in the morning I was happy to transfer his care to the surgical service.

Another patient was an 18-year-old girl, about three months pregnant, who was comatose from a self-administered overdose of an unknown substance. After washing out her stomach to remove whatever was left of the toxic substance, our job was to keep her breathing until the stomach washings could be analyzed and specific treatment started. There was very little time left over to try to comfort her boyfriend, who sat at her bedside throughout the night. Unfortunately, she did not have a good outcome.

A third patient was a comatose man in his early twenties who had a form of meningitis, that is, inflammation of the coverings of the brain and spinal cord. His type of meningitis was caused by spirochetes in his spinal fluid. Spirochetes are the organisms that cause syphilis. I almost got myself into trouble when I informed the patient's significant other, who was present, of the diagnosis. It seemed important to me that she should know about this infectious, sexually transmitted disease so that she could protect herself. Not true. I was given a severe lecture about patient confidentiality by my supervising staff physician. I had no right to give out such information without the patient's consent, he said, and the patient would have every right to sue me for malpractice if and when he recovered. Fortunately, penicillin was effective and available for the treatment of syphilis, and the patient did recover. I felt lucky that the question of a lawsuit was never brought up.

Actually, I was never involved in a lawsuit throughout my entire career of practicing medicine. I carried malpractice insurance, of course, but in those early years pediatricians were considered to be at very low risk for malpractice suits. Our insurance rates were therefore lower than the rates for other specialties. I believe this is no longer true for pediatricians.

THE EMERGENCY ROOM

The month I spent on the emergency service was indeed a busy time. Our working schedule consisted of 24 hours on and 24 hours off. We got no sleep during the 24 hours on, so we had to sleep the first eight and the last eight of the 24 hours off. That left exactly eight hours every other day to take care of our own needs.

One of our duties on the emergency service was to ride the ambulance. Much of the area we covered was in a high crime part of town, but we felt safe because the police usually got to the scene before the ambulance did. Only once did the police fail to be there first for me, and the incident happened when we went out to pick up the victim of a shooting. The ambulance was stopped before we got there by an enormous young black man who was crying, actually blubbering, over a gunshot wound in his arm. He didn't seem very scary, so we took him on board. When we got to the shooting scene, the victim was dead and did not need our services. After we transported our man back to the hospital for treatment, we found out that he was the murderer.

Minneapolis is a city filled with beautiful lakes, and the ambulance was called often in the summer for water emergencies. At least two persons drowned in the lakes each week, and every now and then a toddler would drown in Minnehaha Creek, which was not more than two feet deep. Of the ambulance runs I made that involved drowning, I cannot remember ever resuscitating a single patient. However, when I was a pediatric resident later on, a child who was admitted to the hospital because of near-drowning was successfully treated and did recover. More about that later. In subsequent years the city instituted various programs to teach and publicize water safety, with the result that the number of drownings greatly decreased.

THE BABY JENSEN DEBACLE

My time on the busy pediatric service became busier than ever after the Baby Jensen incident that made headline news across the nation. An investigation by the mayor of Minneapolis, Hubert H. Humphrey, and the Minneapolis Police Department revealed that in the evening of January 12, 1948, Baby Jensen's parents had brought him to the MGH emergency room. He had a chest x-ray that was negative for pneumonia, was treated with a penicillin injection, and the parents were asked to bring him to pediatric clinic in the morning. He was sent home over the objections of his parents, who felt that he should be hospitalized. His condition became worse during the night, and, instead of bringing him back to the hospital, the parents took him in the morning to the office of Mayor Hubert H. Humphrey. Baby Jensen died on the mayor's desk. The pediatric and emergency room residents, who had jointly made the decision to send him home were vilified in the local newspapers, and the story was in every newspaper in the U.S.

After that, every child who came to the MGH emergency room with a sniffle was admitted to the pediatric in-patient service.

SERVICE IN PANAMA

After finishing his internship, Fran was immediately re-inducted into the Army, as pay-back for his medical school years, and was sent through a series of training programs in various places in the United States. He served in Panama during most of the year I spent interning at the MGH, and he ended up writing a book about that year (*Flight Surgeon & Intern*, Noble House, Baltimore, 2005). I was teased a great deal about my absent husband, often at lunch time in the dining room, and usually by our resident surgeons. The men, most of whom had served in the military, had quite a bit to say about how Army personnel behaved, and they told many tales about alcoholism and whoring among men in the service. I, of course, kept quiet, as I had learned to do in medical school. One day the intern with whom I rotated on call took me aside and earnestly informed me that he, for one, did not believe my husband was really drinking and running around with other women in Panama. I thanked him for his kind words, but I was secretly amused because I did not believe it either.

SCANDAL

An incident that happened on Thanksgiving Day might have been a little payback for all the teasing. My brother Al came to the hospital in the afternoon to pick me up and drive me home for Thanksgiving dinner. The receptionist at the nurses' dormitory called me to say that my boyfriend was here for me, and the receptionist at the hospital also called me to say that my husband was here to pick me up. I did not correct either one. Al has blue eyes and blond hair, but I inherited my father's brown eyes and brown hair. As we left the lobby of the hospital, I took his arm to steady myself because the front steps and sidewalk were icy. The next day the hospital's grapevine was full of news about Dr. Haddy's "blonde brother," and the scandal went 'round and 'round. It finally stopped when my friend Elaine McKenzie, who was also interning at the MGH, convinced people that I really did have a blonde brother.

INTERNSHIP COMPLETED

At the end of my year of internship I left the MGH with feelings of relief because those long hours of hard work were over, mixed with sadness because of losing the comradeship that all of us who worked there enjoyed.

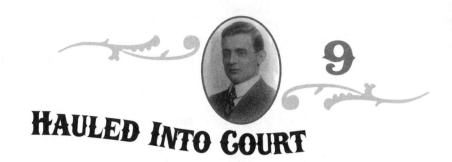

HAULED INTO COURT

efore 1840, medical malpractice was not of serious concern in the United States. After that the numbers of patients who sued their physicians increased each year, and malpractice litigation became a serious issue. It was estimated that by 1850, nine out of every ten physicians in western New York State had been charged with malpractice. In 1885, Henry F. Campbell, in his inaugural speech as president of the American Medical Association, discussed the physician as expert witness as well as confidentiality between patient and physician, but his main concern was about medical malpractice. He called for the establishment of a Section of Medical Jurisprudence within the organization.

Although my father expended a good deal of time and effort upholding the law as Redwood County's coroner, he also had several brushes with the law in which he was the defendant. One of the episodes involved a malpractice issue, and the other two had to do with financial matters.

MALPRACTICE INSURANCE

Although it is not known when he first signed up for medical protective insurance, among his papers is Certificate number 49581 from the Medical Protective Company of Fort Wayne, Indiana [Figures 25a and 25b] indicating that he renewed his contract with the company for April 3, 1928, through April 3, 1929, for an annual premium of $21.00. The original date of the policy is not known. The records relating to his malpractice trial show no evidence that an insurance company was involved in his defense, suggesting that the insurance policy was obtained at a later date. At some point in his career he placed all property, including the family home and his farm, in my mother's name. This was a precaution against malpractice claims, but was also intended to serve as a financial protection for her and their children in the event of his death.

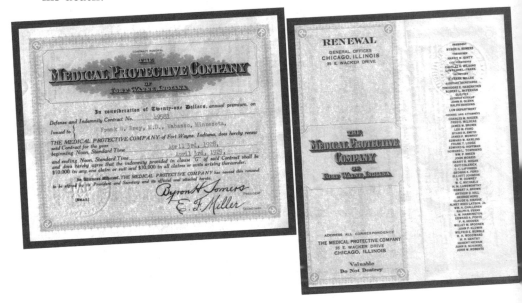

Fig. 25a, b: *Certificate of contract renewal by the Medical Protective Company of Fort Wayne, Indiana, for malpractice insurance covering the period from April 3, 1928, to April 3, 1929.*

MALPRACTICE ACCUSATION

SUMMONS. The Redwood County court records show that on August 17, 1922, Defendant Frank Brey was served a Summons and Complaint by the Sheriff of Redwood County. For performing this duty, Sheriff L. J. Kise was paid $6.00, of which $1.00 was for service and $5.00 for mileage. In the summons, dated the previous day in New Ulm, the State of Minnesota "hereby summoned and required" the defendant to "answer the complaint of the plaintiff...within twenty days."

COMPLAINT. In her complaint filed in the District Court of the Ninth Judicial District of the County of Redwood in the State of Minnesota, which was titled Lorena DeLong, Plaintiff v Frank Brey, Defendant, "Plaintiff complains of defendant and alleges:

"I. That at all times herein mentioned, defendant was and he still is a physician, practising [sic] his profession in the county and state aforesaid.

"II. That on or about the 19th day of October, 1921, plaintiff was pregnant and about to be delivered of a child and then and there employed and hired the defendant herein, to attend her during her impending confinement and that the defendant then and there accepted said employment and undertook as her physician to attend and care for her during her said confinement.

"III. That after defendant had entered upon his said employment and at or about the commencement of parturition but before the complete delivery of said child, the defendant, without cause, negligently, wrongfully, willfully, maliciously and wantonly withdrew from his said employment and abandoned the plaintiff and left her wholly without any medical care or attention during a period of several hours and until another physician summoned by the plaintiff's husband arrived.

"IV. That by reason of the premises and as a result of said negligence and misconduct on the part of the defendant, the child of plaintiff died during birth or shortly thereafter, that plaintiff was thereby greatly injured in her health, sustained great and permanent bodily injury, to her nervous system and reproductive organs and otherwise, and suffered great pain and mental anguish all to her damage in the sum of five thousand dollars ($5,000.00).

"Dated at New Ulm, Minnesota, this 17th day of August, A. D. 1922."

Mueller & Streissguth
Attorneys for Plaintiff
New Ulm, Minnesota

ANSWER. In Dr. Brey's answer to the complaint of Lorena DeLong, "the defendant alleges and shows to the Court:

"I. Defendant admits the allegations of paragraph one.

"II. Further answering, defendant alleges that on or about October 19, 1921, the plaintiff's husband requested the defendant to attend the plaintiff during confinement; that defendant went to plaintiff's home and attempted to comply with the request; but the plaintiff refused to comply with and submit to any of the requirements and precautions of the defendant in the matter of preparing for the child-birth; persistently refused to allow the defendant to perform his tasks according to the usual and accepted practice of medical men on such occasions, and hindered and purposely prevented the defendant from making any progress in arranging for the delivery of the child; that after making every reasonable effort to overcome the said conduct and action of the plaintiff, the defendant advised her that he could not perform the work under such unfavorable circumstance with any hope of a favorable delivery; that her further persistence and hindrance caused the defendant to leave the plaintiff in the care of the husband and a woman who had been called there to attend to her.

"III. The defendant specifically denies that the plaintiff suffered any injury in any manner whatsoever through the actions of this defendant, and, on information and belief, alleges that if she was injured at all, such injury was caused by her own actions, conduct and negligence of other persons contributing thereto.

"IV. Except as herein specifically admitted, explained or qualified the defendant denies each and every allegation, matter and thing, and each and every part thereof in said complaint contained.

"Wherefore, defendant asks judgment that this action be dismissed and for his costs and disbursements herein.

"Dated September 11, 1922."

Albert H. Enersen
Attorney for Defendant
Lamberton, Minnesota

REPLY. The plaintiff was given the opportunity of rebuttal:

"For her reply to the answer of the defendant herein and to the new matter therein contained, plaintiff denies each and every allegation and each and every part thereof, except as the same admits the allegations of her complaint.

"Dated at New Ulm, Minnesota, this 12th day of September, A. D. 1922."

> Mueller & Streissguth
> Attorneys for Plaintiff
> New Ulm, Minnesota

COURT TRIAL. A jury of twelve was selected, from a roster of 18 individuals. Six jurors had been dismissed, the lawyers for the plaintiff and the defendant having challenged three each of the prospective jurors. Retained as members of the jury were B. L. Dudley, Aug Farber, Ole Reierson, Geo Mages, Wm Hasken, C. B. Root, L. H. Mertz, R. H. Byram, C. O. Borg, E. L. Wright, Albert Raddatz, and Ward Baldwin. Dismissed were Anton Pistulka, Mrs. Bess Wilson, E. E. Converse, E. E. Mosier, Geo S. Danis, and A. E. Kuester. On November 16, 1922, the foreman of the jury. C. B. Root, with the other jurors concurring, announced the "verdict for the plaintiff" and assessed her damages in the sum of one thousand dollars."

STIPULATION. Following the verdict, the participants in the trial had an opportunity to appeal, as indicated by their agreement to extend the time for further motions:

"It is hereby stipulated and agreed by and between the parties hereto that the time heretofore granted for the purposes of such motions as either part to the action might desire to make be and hereby is extended to and including February 1st, 1923 in order to give more time to the reporter for the preparation of the testimony in the case, on account of the volume of work already in his office."

> Mueller & Streissguth
> Attorneys for Plaintiff
> Albert H. Enersen
> Attorney for Defendant

ORDER. The request of Frank Brey, the defendant, for a new trial was denied:

"This matter came on to be heard by the Court at Chambers in the ciry of New Ulm, Brown County, Minnesota, on the 16th day of February, 1923, on motion of the defendant, for an order setting aside the verdict and granting a new trial on the grounds stated in Defendant's notice of motion. Albert H. Enersen appeared as attorney for the defendant in support of said motion, and Mueller & Streissguth appeared as attorneys for the plaintiff in opposition thereto.

"After hearing the arguments of counsel and duly considerating [sic] said matter, it is ordered that said motion be and the same is hereby in all things denied.

"Dated at New Ulm, Minnesota, this 16th day of February, A. D. 1923."

J. M. Olson

District Judge

DISMISSAL. The case came to its final conclusion when the lawyers for the plaintiff officially declared that the defendant had paid the judgment against him:

"The claim of the plaintiff herein, having been paid in full, this action is hereby dismissed with prejudice and without costs.

"Dated this 15th day of March, 1923."

Mueller & Streissguth

Attorneys for Plaintiff

New Ulm, Minnesota

Because the actual transcript of the trial is not available, a number of questions remain unanswered. Was there a previous arrangement for obstetrical care? Had the expectant mother received prenatal care? Probably not. It would not have been unusual in those days for a physician to be called after labor was already under way. One would like to know what actual words were said and what actions were taken. For example, what specific "requirements and precautions...in preparing for the childbirth" had the plaintiff "refused to comply with"? What "tasks" did the plaintiff "refuse to allow the defendant to perform"? Did the patient or her husband order Dr. Brey to leave? I had heard about this case on occasion, and I remember being told that the husband had told him to "get out." In which specific ways did the plaintiff "refuse to comply with and submit to any of the requirements and precautions...in preparing for the child-birth"? Did she refuse to allow him to examine her? Why was no outside medical opinion offered about the patient's "injury to her...nervous system and reproductive organs"? And, finally, was there any evidence as to what caused the baby's death? My father appears to have lost his temper and left in response to verbal abuse, and any health care worker who has dealt with an upset patient or an angry family member will be able to empathize with him. He should not have left, however, until another professional person had arrived to take over the case.

The high expectations that people have for favorable outcomes, the perceived affluence of physicians, the willingness of insurance companies to settle out of court, and a contingency fee system that permits lawyers to collect as much as fifty percent of a settlement must all be partly responsible for the large number of malpractice cases that are brought. Certainly, malpractice litigation accounts for part of the financial cost of medical care. Fortunately, I was never involved in a court case, neither as the person sued nor as an expert witness, in more than fifty years of pediatric practice. However, our son was sued for malpractice during his first year of practicing family medicine, and the experience was devastating for him. This was in spite of the fact that the patient was a child that he had never seen. The child was his partner's patient, and all of the members of the medical group were sued because they were partners. There was a great deal of emotional stress involved with the trial itself. In addition, our son was obliged to give a full explanation for the lawsuit every time he applied for a new medical license in a different state.

FINANCIAL MATTERS

Two claims against Dr. Brey, neither of which was contested, resulted in default judgments against him. On October 24, 1932, a default judgment was found in favor of Riggs Optical Company, a Delaware Corporation, for the remainder of a $220.30 bill. He had already paid $154.83 for "goods, wares, and merchandise" purchased from the optical company. The judge ordered a further payment of $70.70, which included the $65.48 remaining on the debt, $.77 interest (6% per annum), $.75 for the cost of affidavits, and a $3.70 clerk's fee. Interestingly, the case was judged by the Honorable Albert H. Enersen, who had been his defense attorney in the malpractice suit. My parents were meticulous about paying their debts, in full and on time. One can speculate that the reason for non-payment of this particular bill was a defect either in the materials or the service rendered by the Riggs Company.

On January 11, 1935, another default judgment against him was found in favor of the Citizens State Bank of Wabasso and the State of Minnesota. The Great Depression was at its height then, and all of the banks in the state were being closed. My father had borrowed $2500.00 from the Wabasso bank and had made two repayments of $30.00 and $25.00 before the banks went out of business. The $2,898.31 that he was ordered to pay to Elmer A. Benson, Commissioner of Banks, and Robert D. Beery, Examiner in Charge of Liquidation, included interest of 8% per annum, together with cost of the action. For the malpractice case his occupation had been listed as "physician," but in this instance, his occupation was, "Has an interest in local grain elevator and oil company."

It was always apparent to me that he greatly distrusted banks. At the time of the Great Depression and the closure of all Minnesota banks, he had lost whatever funds were in his checking and savings accounts. He probably saw no point in sending more of his money into liquidation. We children had each lost small saving accounts of around $10 and $15. When we were invited at a later date to apply for the return of our savings, he commented that it would be a waste of time because there was no likelihood of our ever receiving reimbursement from the bank.

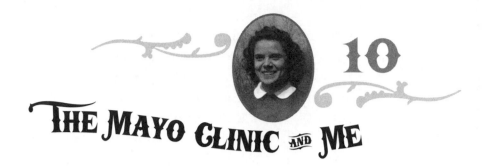

THE MAYO CLINIC AND ME

After completing my internship at the Minneapolis General Hospital (now Hennepin County Medical Center), at the end of June, 1947, I worked part-time as a physician in three not very strenuous jobs: the student health service of the University of Minnesota, the Minneapolis public school system, and in well-baby clinics for the city of Minneapolis. Fran was working on a master's degree in physiology at the University while waiting for his Mayo Clinic fellowship in internal medicine to become available. He had been unexpectedly discharged from the Army in early 1948 (his second discharge from the Army). He had received an acceptance from the Mayo Clinic for an internal medicine fellowship, but because of the large number of returning veterans, an opening for him would not occur for about a year. Residents at the Mayo Clinic were then called fellows.

I applied at the Mayo Clinic for a pediatric fellowship and was accepted for July, 1950, which would be a year later than Fran's starting date of July, 1949. We were delighted. We were expecting our first child around December 25th, and this would give us time to get the baby settled. Rick actually arrived a bit later than we expected.

DUMPED!

A telephone call changed everything. I received a call from Dr. Victor Johnson at the Mayo Clinic, asking me to start in January instead of in July, 1950, because one of the current fellows would be leaving early. I replied that I would like to keep to my scheduled starting date, explained my reason, and thought nothing more about the telephone discussion. A few days later I was surprised and devastated to receive another call from Dr. Victor Johnson, telling me that my acceptance for fellowship was withdrawn and that Mayo would not have a place for me after all. The Mayo Clinic had reneged! The pediatric chairman thought that I should stay home and care for my child. I called back several times, not quite believing what I had heard, but the Mayo Clinic was adamant. The decision was final.

Fran and I were very disappointed to say the least. I felt quite sure that this would not have happened if my father, who customarily referred many of his patients to the Mayo Clinic, had been alive. We considered and dismissed the idea of a legal challenge. Perhaps we should have pursued this option more strongly. First, we had no money to pay a lawyer. In retrospect, we could have borrowed money. Second, we had never heard of the Mayo Clinic losing a lawsuit. We did not realize then that the Mayo Clinic settles suits out of court from time to time. Third, even though I surely would have been reinstated if I had pursued the matter legally, the reputation of trouble-maker would have followed me throughout my time at the Mayo Clinic. It also would have reflected badly on Fran.

ROCHESTER

Fran obtained his master's degree in physiology at the University of Minnesota, and we moved to Rochester so that Fran could start his residency on July 1, 1949. Rick was born in St. Marys Hospital on January 8, 1950, in the middle of a big snowstorm. In those days the Mayo Clinic kept first-time mothers and infants in the hospital for a full week. We took him home to the duplex we lived in, and he turned out to be very easy to care for; he never cried, slept like an angel, and performed all of his developmental milestones right on time. We took all of that for granted and assumed that we must be good parents to have such a well behaved baby.

RESIDENCY

Since my plan to train in pediatrics at the Mayo Clinic had not worked out, I applied to the Minneapolis General Hospital, which was controlled by the University of Minnesota, and I felt fortunate to be accepted by the Department of Pediatrics. The MGH hospital director gave me a good recommendation, and I ended up serving a pediatric residency at the University of Minnesota, with most of my time spent at the Minneapolis General Hospital, from July 1, 1950, to June 30, 1952.

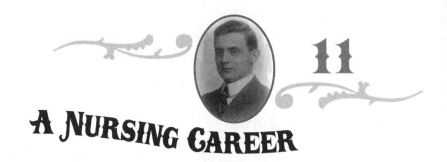

A NURSING CAREER

After the distinguished British nurse, Florence Nightingale, published her Notes on Nursing in England in 1860, greater respect began to develop for nursing as a profession. A nursing association and a nursing journal were established. Groups of nurses organized and pressured legislatures to pass nurse registration laws. Nurses' training was customarily provided by hospitals, but the University of Minnesota gave academic credence to the profession in 1909 by establishing a three-year program leading to a nursing diploma. In 1947, a five-year program that led to a bachelor of science degree was established. Prior to the nineteenth century, the management of mentally ill patients was characterized by cruelty and neglect, but by the early 1800s, this kind of treatment was being replaced by "moral treatment," a kinder, gentler form of therapy. By the mid-nineteenth century, many state hospitals, called insane asylums, had been established for taking care of psychotic patients. Then, in 1900, Sigmund Freud published The Interpretation of Dreams in Austria and introduced a new way of thinking about the treatment of neuroses.

While my father was beginning his medical practice in Wabasso, my mother was growing up on the Daub family farm two miles north of town. Whether they had ever met is not known, but she must have been aware of him. When my mother left home in 1911 to begin training as a nurse at the Rochester State Hospital, my father had been practicing medicine in Wabasso for a year.

ELIZABETH DAUB

Elizabeth Katherine Daub was born on September 1, 1892, thirty years after the Sioux Uprising of 1862, on the family farm in Vail township. The village of Wabasso had not yet been established. The second child born to her parents, she was delivered at home by my mother's Aunt Lizzie. At 19 years of age she traveled with her trunk by train to Rochester, Minnesota, where she enrolled in the Rochester State Hospital School of Nursing. In those days, using a trunk as a form of heavy baggage was not unusual, and her trunk, which was always very private, remained important to her. It still resides in the attic of my family home. My father had his own trunk, too, and it resides in the attic alongside my mother's trunk. Although Elizabeth (nobody ever called her Betty) did not know what a nurse was or what a nurse did, her ambition, as long as she could remember, had been to be a nurse. When she set out to accomplish this aim, she had never seen a nurse, nor attended high school, nor traveled away from her farm home. "The weather was very cold that year," my Uncle Robert Daub remembered, "twenty, thirty, forty degrees below zero all winter long, one of the coldest winters we ever had."

IMMIGRATION

My mother's parents [Figure 26] came to Minnesota, as did my father's parents, with the wave of German-speaking immigrants who arrived while the Minnesota River Valley, including most of the lower one-third of the state, was recovering from the devastation that followed the Sioux Uprising of 1862. "Free land in America" was being advertised in Germany. The would-be immigrants were told that they would find the new land "flowing with milk and honey," and even though the people surely did not take the words literally, their expectations must have been high. I often heard my mother use the phrase when telling us children why her family came to America.

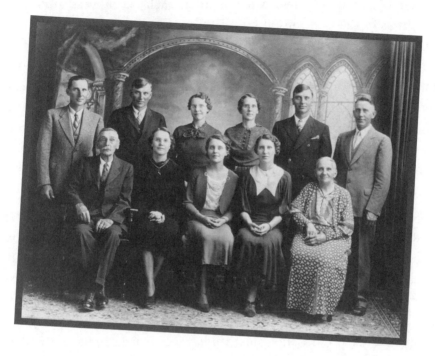

Fig. 26: *Photograph of the Daub family circa 1935. Front row, seated, from left, John Evangelist Daub II, Therese, Helen, Anne, and Katherine Zeug Daub. Back row, standing, from left, Ludwig, Joseph, Clara, Elizabeth, Robert, and John.*

White Settlers

The first white settlers arrived in Redwood County, still further up the river and to the north and west of Brown County, a few years later. The northeastern border of Redwood County was formed by the great Minnesota River. Two major rivers, the Redwood in the north and the Cottonwood in the south, which flowed into the Minnesota River, bordered the central portion of the county, the last portion of the county to be settled and where the village of Wabasso would be placed. A number of creeks contributed to the rivers and a small lake on the land that was homesteaded by my great-grandfather Daub. The flat land was covered with tallgrass that in turn covered a deep layer of dark topsoil. Layers of grass had pressed down upon each other, year after year, resulting in the rich topsoil found throughout the Great Plains. As a result, grain grew abundantly and agriculture in the area was one of the most productive, if not the most productive, in the nation. Of the few trees that were present, willows and cottonwoods predominated, except for a few oak and maple trees. In the southwest corner of Redwood County, a large grove of black walnut trees grew near Plum Creek, which emptied into the Cottonwood River and about which Laura Ingalls Wilder wrote her charming stories. The town of Walnut Grove later became established at this site.

Andrew Koch and his wife were the first settlers to take up a claim in Redwood County, when they moved into the grove of black walnut trees located near Plum Creek in 1857. Redwood County was created by the state legislature in 1862; until then the area was simply Minnesota Territory. A stockade was built at Redwood Falls in 1864. Although the Indian uprising began and ended in 1862, the stockade was thought to be needed for protection against raids by renegade Indians. Dr. D. L. Hitchcock, who arrived in Redwood Falls in 1865, became the first physician and pharmacist in Redwood County. (In those days, physicians frequently dispensed their own drugs because of the dearth of pharmacists who could fill their prescriptions.)

AFTERMATH OF THE 1862 UPRISING

Most of the Indians had been banished from Minnesota, but a residue of unease and anger remained among the whites. So many people had been killed or had fled from the area that the entire upper Minnesota River Valley, a tract of land two hundred miles long by fifty or more miles wide, including 23 counties, was almost entirely depopulated. The greatest loss of life from the conflict had occurred among the German settlers in Renville and Brown Counties. The killing did not end with the executions at Mankato. Chief Little Crow returned to Minnesota in 1863, and several murders took place in Kandiyohi, Wright, and Stearns Counties, in areas where the chief and his band of warriors were known to have been present. It was never known for sure, however, that they were guilty of these murders. Little Crow was killed on July 3, 1863, in McLeod County after exchanging shots with a father and son who came upon him while hunting. Probably the last Indian ambush in Minnesota occurred in 1865 when four members of the Andrew Jewett family were murdered by Indians in Blue Earth County near Mankato. Although Minnesota was quiet after that, the Indian wars were continuing in the states to which the Sioux had fled, and the immigrants could not be confident that there would be no further uprisings in Minnesota. One can imagine how the children, especially those living on lonely farms across the lower third of the state of Minnesota, must have been terrified of going to sleep some nights, thinking about tales they had heard of children being scalped or kidnapped.

THE HOMESTEAD ACT

According to the Minnesota Homestead Act of 1862, any head of family who was over 21 years of age could claim up to a quarter section, that is, 160 acres, of public land. If the settler resided on the land for five continuous years and improved the land, the government granted free title to the tract. "Improvement" meant to build a house and cultivate the land, and when the farmer went to the land office to prove that the requirements had been met, it was called "proving up." The claimant could be absent from the land for as long as six months without losing his claim.

THE ZEUG FAMILY

My mother's mother, Katherine Zeug, was a three-year-old child when she and her mother, Anna Liebl Zeug, came to join her father in New Ulm in 1868. It was six years after the Sioux Uprising and three yeas after the end of the Civil War. She was born in Prague on January 1, 1864, in what later became the Czech Republic, of an ethnic German family. Two infant siblings had died on the difficult sea voyage to New York. Her father, John Baptiste Zeug, who had arrived in the United States the year before, first worked in a mill but later owned and operated a combination home-store-bar on Minnesota Street in New Ulm. He was an accomplished musician who also organized a band and gave music lessons on the violin. In 1876, or possibly 1877, he staked out a homestead near Walnut Grove. He dug a shelter in a hill, a prairie sod house, where he lived while establishing the homestead, and he moved his family there the following year. The farm grew several crops, but the main one was wheat, which had to be hauled to Walnut Grove to sell. When the Cottonwood River was so high that he could not cross it, he hauled his wheat instead to Marshall. Later John Baptiste built a large house for his growing family, a house that is still owned and lived in on the original homestead by a member of the Zeug family.

Eventually Anna and John had 13 more children, to a total of 16. Two more died in infancy, and the 12 who survived were Katherine, John Baptist, Frank, Mary, Emma, Joseph, Otto, Rose (Sister Rudolphina), Anna (Sister Sidonia), Elizabeth (Sister Irmengard), Louise (Sister Stephen), and Paul. Of the four girls who became Benedictine nuns, three remained in the convent throughout their lives, while the fourth, Louise, left the convent for a secular career. The nuns were highly respected in my family. A photograph of the four in their black habits, along with their mother, also dressed in black, none of them smiling, hung in my bedroom when I was a child. Those black robes and sober faces, to me somewhat reminiscent of a row of black crows, were scary. They seemed to brood over me as I fell asleep every night. I'm sure those kind, gentle ladies, as I learned to know them in later years, would have been sad to hear that they had frightened a small child. Katherine Zeug Daub died on December 4, 1939.

THE DAUB FAMILY

My mother's grandfather, John Evangelist Daub, emigrated from Heidelberg, western Germany, where he became one of the earliest settlers in Redwood County. In 1871 he established a homestead in Vail

Township, two miles north of where the village of Wabasso would later arise. Born on December 31, 1812, he attained a college education in Germany, and he had been teaching school for 30 years before he decided to emigrate. He and his wife had married in 1842, and their children were Theodore, Elizabeth, Ellinore, John Evangelist II (my grandfather, born on January 4, 1856), Matilda, and Amelia.

My grandfather's older brother, Theodore, who was born in Wurtemburg, Germany, on November 4, 1844, came to the United States in May, 1870. According to my Uncle Louie Daub, Theodore left Germany before the rest of the family to avoid serving in the Austro-Hungarian army, with the intention of acquiring land of his own. My Great Uncle Theodore located first in Iowa, subsequently moved to New Ulm, and then worked for a time on a farm near Redwood Falls. He probably decided to homestead at the same time my great-grandfather did, in 1871, each taking a quarter section of land. Theodore lived with his wife, Helen Augusta (Aunt 'Gusta) Feige, and family on the neighboring farm for many years. He was active in community affairs, having been elected at the first meeting of the residents of Vail Township in 1879 to serve as one of the township's first two justices. (The other was John Taber, Wabasso's first settler, who had arrived two years earlier, in 1869.)

There were no trees on the prairie homestead and therefore no wood with which to build a house. According to Uncle Louie Daub, the sod house was dug into a hill located between the previous site of the one-room schoolhouse (District 60) and where the barn is now. After living for two years in the sod house, they fetched lumber from the Redwood Falls area, made from trees that grew near the river, and built a house. Theodore owned ten acres of land near the Redwood River, which furnished wood for building and also fuel for both of the Daub families.

SOD HOUSES

Many of the early settlers who homesteaded in the interior of Redwood County had no choice but to build sod houses because no trees were immediately available for wood. The densely packed roots and root hairs of the tallgrasses formed a sod from ten to twelve inches deep, which could be cut and used like bricks. Actually, the sod was so thick and firm that it could not be plowed under by an ordinary team of horses with a plow; oxen were required to pull the plowshare when the land was first plowed. According to some estimates, ninety percent of the settlers built their first homes with these three-foot long sod bricks. Precise instruction for building a sod house is furnished by Everett Dick in his description of how to build "a rather pretentious sod house" in *The Best of the West*, edited by Tony Hillerman, HarperCollins, New York, 1991. In contrast to laying the foundation on flat Kansas land, with four walls and the roof of sod, as Dick described, my relatives were more likely to build on a hillside and dig part way into the earth, so that three walls were of dirt and only the front wall and roof were of sod.

My cousin Ambrose (Andy) Schmelzle's wife, Myrtle, described her maternal grandmother's early years, which included living in a sod house: "My mother's mother, Myrtle Knight, homesteaded with her family south of Wabasso. She lived in a sod hut for the first year or so—she remembered this very well. Mounds of dirt are still present at the sites of the original sod huts near the Cottonwood River, so that we know exactly where the homes were. She married into the Cantine family. They were farmers, and they farmed a large acreage in the Walnut Grove area. Plum Creek ran through the Cantine farm, and their land was adjacent to the farm where the Ingalls family lived for a year. The Cantine girls played with the Ingalls girls. Laura Ingalls Wilder later wrote the *Little House on the Prairie* series of children's books."

In her book, *On the Banks of Plum Creek*, Harper & Row, New York, 1937, Laura Ingalls Wilder told about the sod house she lived in, a dugout in one of the banks of Plum Creek. She first described the stable, "Grass grew on its walls and its roof was covered with growing grasses, blowing in the wind." Of the house itself, she wrote, "The one-room interior had smooth, hard earth walls that had been whitewashed. The smooth, hard floor was earth, too. The front wall was built of sod, with a small greased-paper window beside the door. Willow boughs, their branches woven together, formed the ceiling, and grass grew on the roof, waving in the wind just like all the grasses along the creek bank."

THE GRASSHOPPER PLAGUE

The early years when the grasshoppers denuded the countryside must have been a terrible time for the settlers, who were just getting started. The grasshopper invasion was at its worst from 1873 to 1876. The insects came in such swarms that they looked like a dust storm, blotting out the sun. My mother spoke of hearing about the "plague of locusts" from family members. Uncle Louie Daub recalled that he was told how the chickens ate so many live grasshoppers that the egg yolks turned red and were inedible. "The grasshoppers were dried and fed to the chickens in small amounts, as a supplement, during the winter," he said. "Also, in winter the farmers ate a soup made from the dried grasshoppers, a broth that was drained from the grasshoppers."

TYPHOID FEVER

Other difficulties that the new farmers faced were prairie fires and, in winter, blizzards. Illness was the worst problem of all, however, and the Daub family suffered severely when my great-grandmother and great-aunt Amelia died of typhoid fever contracted by drinking water from a shallow well near the farm. Because there were no cemeteries, they were buried in a small plot on their own land. My great-grandfather was eventually laid to rest there too. The Daub homestead is still occupied by a family member, and the graveyard, with its single tombstone and three small markers, remains exactly as it was a century ago. Near the small cemetery, a patch of original prairie grass has been preserved. An anecdote, which circulated within the family for many years, asserted that Great Aunt 'Gusta had planted poison ivy on the graves. According to my mother, Augusta was not affected by the plant's toxin and thought the leaves of the plant pretty. It seems more likely to me, however, that the story reflected how people felt about Aunt 'Gusta!

THE HOMESTEAD

John Evangelist Daub II and Katherine Zeug were married in John-
sonville Township on May 25, 1886. Because my grandfather was not
the oldest son, he would not ordinarily have been the one to manage the
family property. His only brother, Theodore, was already settled on the
adjoining farm, however, so John Evangelist inherited the homestead.
John and Katherine had nine children who lived, and a tenth child who
died as a newborn. John Evangelist Daub died on October 18, 1948.

ELIZABETH'S EARLY SCHOOLING

My mother grew up on the farm [Figure 27] with her four sisters
and four brothers [Figure 26], and she completed the eighth grade at the
one-room schoolhouse situated on the edge of the farmland. Her diploma
[Figure 28], dated June 16, 1906, certified that "Lizzie Daub, a student
of this school, who has secured an attendance mark of 75% during this
school year, and during this period has fully complied with all rules
and regulations of the school known as District No. 60 is given this
Diploma for excellent work, for punctuality, and for good deportment
during such attendance." The diploma was signed by Nellie F. Hender-
son, Teacher, and by P. J. Race, the (Redwood) County superintendent
of schools. At the time my mother was graduating from the eighth

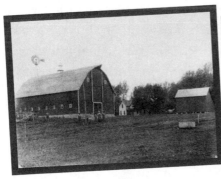
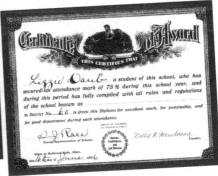

(From Left To Right)
Fig. 27: *An early photograph of the Daub farm home.*

Fig. 28: *Lizzie Daub's elementary school diploma from School District 60,
June 16, 1906.*

grade, my father was completing his first academic year at the University of Minnesota. Because Wabasso had only recently been founded (in 1900), there was no high school for her to attend when she completed elementary school.

HER SIBLINGS

Elizabeth's sister Clara, and her brothers Joseph, Ludwig, and John were not able to attend high school either, although Joe took a business school course in Mankato and Clara enrolled in a nurses' training course in Mercy Hospital, Devil's Lake, North Dakota. Clara's training was cut short because of illness. Therese, Anne, and Helen were sent to St. Benedict's boarding school in St. Cloud after they completed the eighth grade. Anne and Helen returned home to attend the local high school after it opened, with Anne finishing in the first graduating class of 1919, and Helen finishing in 1923. Robert spent four years in the Wabasso Public High School and graduated in 1928. Anne and Therese became school teachers, Helen became an occupational therapist, and Clara, who had been forced to give up her nursing career because of illness, became a housewife. All four of the boys became independent farmers. It has always seemed interesting to me that in my mother's family the girls became educated and the boys received land.

THE ROCHESTER STATE HOSPITAL

I remember that my mother talked a lot to us children about how nurses in training were treated in those days. Student nurses worked fourteen hours every day, seven days each week, she said. Their duties included scrubbing floors and cooking for their patients. Student nurses were not allowed to wear makeup and were closely chaperoned. They were not expected to date, and the idea of a student nurse being married was unheard of. Only after working a full year were they permitted to return to their homes for a first visit. Nursing tended to follow the pattern set up by Florence Nightingale, with strong emphasis upon loyalty to the profession. Strict discipline whether on duty or not, long hours, hard work, and low pay were all taken for granted.

Although the hospital had no formal affiliation with the Mayo Clinic, student nurses who became ill received their medical care at the Clinic. My mother often mentioned, with pride, that her medical record at the Mayo Clinic was established during her student days.

In becoming a psychiatric nurse (as would naturally follow since she was trained in a psychiatric hospital) she learned how to deal with mentally ill patients who sometimes became hostile and combative. Because modern tranquilizers and psychotropic drugs were not available, nurses and orderlies in mental hospitals utilized other methods of treatment, including sedatives, hydrotherapy, and in extreme instances, restraints and padded rooms. Occupational therapy was available in mental institutions (Aunt Helen Daub studied occupational therapy in college), but it was not until later that various forms of counseling and psychotherapy were routinely integrated into the patients' treatment plans.

GRADUATION

My mother's class of six women and one man graduated from nursing school in 1914. The exercise was held in the Amusement Hall of the hospital, and the invitation [Figures 29a and 29b] to the twenty-third annual commencement of the Rochester State Hospital Training School for Nurses lists the other graduates as Florence Montgomery, Cora Elizabeth Diegnau, Emma Rose Schoeb, Mary O'Brien, Tora Anderson, and J. H. Kirkham. The diplomas were presented by Dr. Arthur F. Kilbourne, the hospital director, and the address was given by Dr. O. C. Heyerdale, the assistant director. My mother's diploma [Figure 30] certified that "Elizabeth Kathrine [sic] Daub has completed with credit a three years' course of instruction and practical training in this Institution…on June 15, 1914." She was now allowed to wear a thin black ribbon on her nursing cap, signifying that she was no longer a student but now a graduate nurse [Figures 31 and 32]. After passing a written examination, she became registered nurse number 2,035 in Minnesota. At that time, nurses' registration in the state was for life, and no renewal was required. The man in the class went on to become a hos-

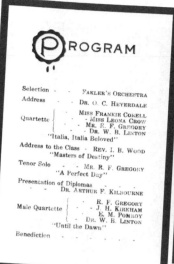

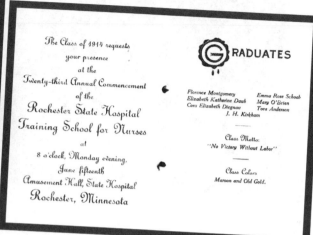

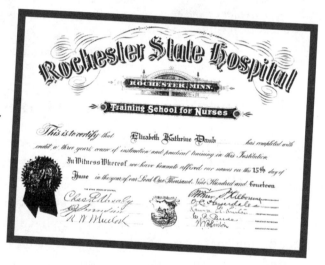

(Clockwise From Top Left)

Fig. 29a,b: *Invitation by the Class of 1914 to the Twenty-third Annual Commencement of the Rochester State Hospital Training School for Nurses, Rochester, Minnesota, on June 15, 1914.*

Fig. 30: *Elizabeth Kathrine [sic] Daub's certificate of graduation from the Rochester State Hospital Training School for Nurses, June 15, 1914.*

pital administrator; this was not an unusual route in those days to train for hospital administration.

My mother treasured her nursing textbooks and carefully preserved them. Among her books that remain in the library of my family home are: *Text-Book of Anatomy and Physiology for Nurses, Primary Studies for Nurses: a Text-Book for First Year Pupil Nurses, Clinical Studies for Nurses: a Text-Book for Second and Third Year Pupil Nurses, A Nurse's Handbook of Obstetrics,* and *Modern Methods of Nursing.*

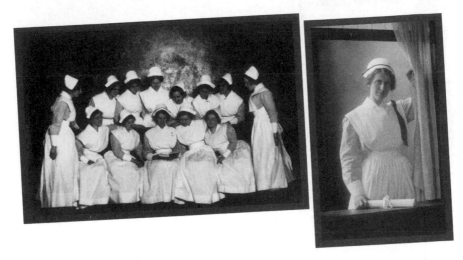

(From Left To Right)
Fig. 31: *A group of nurses. Elizabeth Katherine Daub, in the center, is the only one who has a black band on her cap, signifying that she has graduated from her training course.*

Fig. 32: *Elizabeth Katherine Daub, with her diploma and a new black band across her cap, at graduation from nurses' training.*

THE MINNEAPOLIS GENERAL HOSPITAL

After working for a time as a private duty psychiatric nurse at the Rochester State Hospital, Elizabeth went to the Minneapolis General Hospital [Figure 33] for a year-long postgraduate course in infectious diseases. She and her classmates lived in the hospital annex—they called it "the pesthouse"—and she may have had a bout with diphtheria during that year. All of the patients who had infections were collected in the annex building, which was separated from the main hospital by a courtyard. Members of the nursing staff lived in the annex and were not allowed to leave the building for fear of spreading disease, but those who were adventuresome would sneak out at night for a walk around the city block. If one considers that no specific treatment was available for any of the infectious diseases, and that only prevention was effective, it is not difficult to understand why measures were employed that would be considered extreme by today's standards. The annex was later used for pediatric and psychiatric patients, and patients

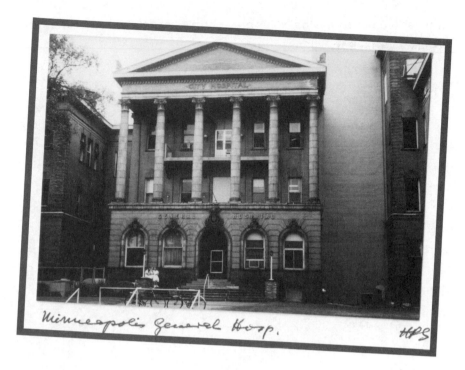

Fig. 33: *The Minneapolis General Hospital. From the collection of Dr. and Mrs. Henry P. Staub.*

with infectious diseases, regardless of age, continued to be housed there. It had its own outpatient area, as well. The annex of the Minneapolis General Hospital provided an important part of my training during my years as a medical student, intern, and pediatric resident at the University of Minnesota. All acute phase poliomyelitis patients who came to the hospital during the 1946 poliomyelitis epidemic were first seen there as outpatients. Those who were diagnosed to have poliomyelitis were admitted to hospital beds in the annex wards.

"She was next employed as charge nurse in Cottage 8 at the Anoka State Hospital," said Uncle Robert, "where she developed a kidney infection and was sent home to rest. She was slated to be the charge nurse at the new Glen Lake Tuberculosis Sanitarium. The 1918 flu epidemic came along, however, and she decided instead to stay at home and help out as best she could." After the flu epidemic was over, my father asked her to stay on as his office nurse, and they were married on November 24, 1921, Thanksgiving Day.

THE LATER YEARS

My mother loved her work, and she often talked to us children about her nursing studies and her work as a graduate nurse. In fact, she frequently expressed the hope that she could some day return to hospital nursing, and, as it happened, she eventually did. After my father's death, she took a refresher course in nursing at the University of Minnesota during the years of the Second World War, while I was a medical student there. She did this at a time when it was very unusual for older students to attend the University. She returned to psychiatric nursing at the St. Cloud Veterans' Hospital and worked there until she retired.

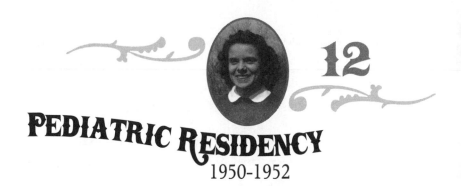

PEDIATRIC RESIDENCY
1950-1952

I returned to the Minneapolis General Hospital as a pediatric resident on July 1, 1950. My mother had agreed that I could live with
her and my siblings in the family home, the Red House in St. Paul,
and she would care for our son Rick while I completed my two year
pediatric residency. Our son Rick was six months old when I began my
residency and two-and-one-half years old when I finished. All of the
family members loved him. With my mother in charge, I never had to
worry about his welfare. He was a bright, appealing baby and toddler
who never cried, and we watched his development with interest and
amazement. As he learned to talk, his use of words and phrases was
especially intriguing. We still use the word "cuppee," for "cup of coffee," and "nean," for "neat and clean."

Fran, who by then had completed six months of his internal medicine training at the Mayo Clinic, remained in Rochester. He lived at the
Wilson Club, a house for single Mayo men, and commuted to St. Paul
twice weekly to be with Rick and me. He never once failed to make the
trip on Wednesday or Thursday nights and the weekend, no matter
how severe the Minnesota winter weather.

MAYO CLINIC POSTSCRIPT

There was a postscript to my story about the Mayo Clinic: a few
months after I began my residency at the University, Fran received a

telephone call asking if I were available, because a place had opened up in the Department of Pediatrics.

MINNEAPOLIS GENERAL HOSPITAL

As a pediatric resident I stayed at the hospital to take night calls approximately every third night; we were paid $100 each month. Norman Sterrie and Henry Staub, who were pediatric residents around the same time I was, were good friends and especially helpful to me. Although we were University of Minnesota pediatric residents, we were assigned to and spent most of our time at the Minneapolis General Hospital, serving only brief periods in the pediatric department of the University of Minnesota Hospitals. The work at MGH was interesting, my fellow residents were supportive, and in general things went along smoothly. The only disappointing note was the attitude of most of our U of M based supervising pediatricians. The MGH pediatric service was administered academically by the University of Minnesota. Members of the academic staff routinely made teaching rounds with us at MGH, and at least one of our rotations was through the U of M pediatric hospital service (we also rotated through the St. Mary's Hospital pediatric service). Some of the practicing physicians in Minneapolis, who had clinical appointments at the U of M, also made teaching rounds with us. One of our attending physicians who was outstanding in every way was Dr. Tague Chisholm, who was practicing pediatric surgery in Minneapolis; we could turn to him for surgical problems with confidence that our patient would be treated with skill and compassion and that we would be treated with courtesy.

The U of M instructors tended to be resentful at having to make the trip downtown as well as supercilious about what they perceived as inferior quality of care at MGH, and it was obvious that they looked down on us. When we rotated through the U of M service, we were pretty much treated the same way there.

While I was a pediatric resident I published my first article in which I was the first author. The individual who writes the paper is customarily the first author, with others who have contributed to the work having their names included as second, third, etc. authors. The paper was a review of breast feeding[8], and the U of M attending pediatrician who was supervising the service allowed me to include his name as the second author.

A COUPLE OF GOOD OUTCOMES

On one occasion, I was up all night long at MGH treating a child who had arrived during the evening, comatose, febrile, and very toxic-appearing from Hemophilus influenza bacterial meningitis. Working alone, I inserted an intravenous line and started her on antibiotic therapy. After some hours had gone by without improvement, I telephoned the Public Health Department and requested an antibody preparation, which before the advent of antibiotics had been the only available treatment for H influenza infections. Antibiotics, at this time, were still relatively new. The public health official whose sleep was disturbed was most gracious and sent the material over by courier. The child noticeably improved after it was administered, and by morning she was awake, drinking fluids, and cheerfully greeting everybody who came into her room. Imagine my surprise and dismay when, instead of the expected compliment on doing a good job when the patient was presented at morning rounds, I was roundly excoriated by the U of M attending pediatrician. "Everybody knew," according to him, that antibiotic therapy was sufficient and that giving additional antibody therapy was "out of date." He was correct in that antibiotics alone eventually became the treatment of choice for this disease, but this had not yet become standard medical practice. He was not there during the night, and he had no knowledge of how sick the child was before the antibody was administered. Bacterial meningitis is a uniformly fatal disease if untreated, and it can still be fatal on occasion, even when optimal treatment is given. He should have acknowledged that the additional treatment with antibody did no harm and might have done some good. He was very wrong to publicly disparage another physician, especially one in a subordinate position, in such a ruthless way. This incident helps to illustrate why my feelings toward my alma mater lack warmth.

Another evening one of the MGH residents brought his little daughter, about five years old, into the hospital in a comatose state. The pupils of her eyes were widely dilated. She had no fever and it was quickly determined by a negative spinal tap that she did not have meningitis. A different U of M supervisor, who was on call that night, came to see her at my request, but we all remained puzzled as to what could be the problem. She had been started on an antibiotic for an upper respiratory infection earlier in the day. In order to offer the distraught father a way to help, I asked him to go to the drug store in the Minneapolis suburb where the drug had been obtained and check on the prescription. He came back with the information that the liquid preparation given to her mistakenly contained atropine, a drug routinely used in eye drops to dilate the pupils in order to make it easier to examine the eyes. The information enabled us to start specific therapy, and the child recovered without any adverse side effects.

NEAR-DROWNING

A ten-year-old girl was brought in to the MGH by ambulance in July, 1951, in great distress because of difficulty breathing. She had been resuscitated after being immersed in one of the Minneapolis freshwater lakes for two to three minutes. Her problem was pulmonary edema, which improved after several days of treatment with positive pressure oxygen. Fortunately, the child did not develop pneumonia. Pulmonary edema, which occurs when the lungs are overloaded with fluid, causes severe difficulty with breathing. This condition, resulting from near-drowning, was just beginning to be recognized, and a few case reports had recently appeared in the medical literature. It formed the basis for the second publication of which I was the first author.[9]

INSUBORDINATION

I managed to get myself in trouble on one occasion. The U of M pediatrics department was negotiating with an out-of-town hospital to rotate pediatric residents through their pediatric service. Most likely this would have supplied a needed service to the other hospital while benefiting the U of M financially. The matter was brought up at a combined meeting with the MGH and U of M residents. An out-of-town rotation was not included in my contract when I accepted the residency position, and it would have been difficult for me to either leave Rick behind in the care of my mother or take my baby with me. The next day I went to the MGH director, a physician with whom I had had a good relationship when I was an intern, and told him that I had a small baby and had no intention of living out of town for any period of time. It was a mistake to have mentioned the baby. Women were not supposed to let their domestic affairs interfere with their work. I should have said that an out-of-town rotation was not included in my original contract. Also, I probably should have talked first to the director of pediatrics before going to the hospital director. The out-of-town rotation never materialized, but I believe this incident of insubordination was held against me from then on.

UNIVERSITY OF MINNESOTA ROTATION

A couple of unusual patients whom I saw while rotating through the U of M service improved my self-esteem to some extent. One was a small boy who came in with eczema covering his entire body, which was overlaid with an extensive purulent exudate, that is, covered with pus. The case was puzzling because all cultures for bacteria were negative. I suggested checking for the vaccinia virus used to vaccinate against smallpox. It turned out that he was infected with the virus from his foster mother, who had recently been vaccinated because she was planning to take a trip abroad. The outcome was, unfortunately, fatal. The other case was a baby with known adrenocorticotropic hormone (ACTH, a hormone produced by the pituitary gland) deficiency who was Dr. Irvine McQuarrie's private patient. Dr. McQuarrie, chairman of the department, was a renowned pediatric endocrinologist. I was the resident who saw the infant upon admission, and, knowing that patients with that diagnosis are prone to suddenly going into shock, I suggested that an intravenous line should be placed immediately even though he appeared normal on physical examination. Dr. McQuarrie declined my suggestion. Within a few hours the baby went into shock with a blood pressure that fell to zero, and he required resuscitation. With the help of my fellow residents, I instituted treatment and the patient did well. I believe this incident was responsible for the very positive letter of reference that Dr. McQuarrie wrote for me a few years later.

U OF M ATTITUDE

The adversarial attitude of the U of M attending staff toward us trainees surely caused resentment among us pediatricians-in-training, who should later have been a source of patient referrals. I had observed the same attitude toward referring physicians throughout my student days. Patients who were sent to the university hospitals by their local physicians (derisively referred to as LMDs) were frequently held up at conferences as examples of incompetence on the part of the LMDs. These, I believe are two very good reasons why the school of medicine at the U of M gradually lost patients and eventually lost its university hospital. Former students and residents as well as outside pediatricians who needed help were treated with disrespect and thus discouraged from making referrals. In addition, such treatment discouraged alumni such as myself from giving financial contributions later. The U of M attitude is in direct contrast to the policy of the Mayo Clinic, where referring and visiting physicians (but not always aspiring residents or fellows) are treated with courtesy.

REFERENCES

8. Haddy, T. B., Adams, F. H. Factors of importance in breast milk. *J Pediatr 40:243-253, 1952.*

9. Haddy, T. B., Disenhouse, R. B. Acute pulmonary edema due to near-drowning in fresh water: case report. *J Pediatr 44:565-569, 1954.*

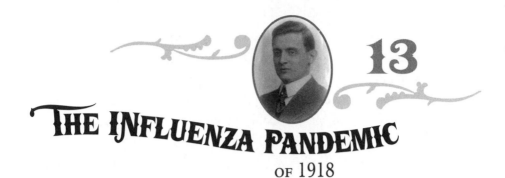

THE INFLUENZA PANDEMIC
OF 1918

*I*n the United States, almost 550,000 persons died in the great influenza pandemic of 1918, five times the number killed in all of the battles of the First World War, which was being fought on European soil. Worldwide, more than one billion persons became ill, and the number of deaths was approximately 25 million. A few scientists had begun to suspect that a virus, rather than a bacillus, was the causative agent. No specific treatment was available for the influenza or its complications.

The influenza epidemic of 1918 was the most disastrous outbreak in American history and the most deadly epidemic that the world had experienced since the bubonic plague in the thirteenth century. This virulent disease, with its serious complications, mainly influenza-pneumonia and influenza-encephalitis, was puzzling in many ways, and much about it remains a mystery to this day. The reasons why it was such a vicious infection—why the death rate was so high, why affected patients succumbed so rapidly, and why the disease spread so rapidly throughout the world—are still unexplained.

Yet, in spite of the tragedy and sadness it caused, the flu of 1918 had a special, tender meaning for my family. Wabasso was more fortunate than many communities because Dr. Brey, the only physician serving the area, was not drafted by the military. My mother was recuperating at home on the Daub family farm from an illness, and she decided to stay on and help care for the sick. My parents-to-be must have worked together on many cases during that calamitous time. According to Uncle Robert Daub, this was probably when the romance began between my father and mother.

My cousin Beatrice Fixsen Emmerick agreed with Uncle Robert: "I remember how Elizabeth was your father's 'right hand man.' She checked on patients who were sick but whose condition was not life threatening. I know she came to see me and I suppose she gave my folks some instructions on caring for me. I know that they worked together constantly. The epidemic was a frightening thing, and I'm sure it was during that time they really got to know one another and the practice and other events that followed. After things got back to normal, I believe, that was when they became serious about each other."

EPIDEMIOLOGY

Because the flu of 1918 attacked not only regions but continents, it became a pandemic. By definition, an epidemic affects many people in a community or region at one time, and an epidemic becomes a pandemic when many cases occur throughout the world within a short period of time. Influenza first appeared in the United States among army recruits, and it probably came to France with the American soldiers who disembarked there, but there is some question that it might have gone the other way. It may have been already present in the ports of Europe and transferred from there to the United States. It spread to England and Spain, increasing in virulence as it went, and became known as "the Spanish flu" or "the Spanish lady" because it caused the death of many Spaniards. It spread devastation throughout the rest of the world and added to the havoc already being caused by the war. It kept the English soldiers from their ranks and the sailors from their ships. It raced through the German army, which was already close to being crushed, and spread across the continent of Europe, attacking

Russia, China, Japan, and India before moving on to the continents of Africa and South America.

The army of the United States, made up of almost two million men, was being mobilized. It is generally believed that the first cases in the United States appeared in Fort Riley, Kansas, on March 11, 1918. One week later, an explosive epidemic of influenza was reported from Fort Ogelthorpe, Tennessee. The infection spread quickly and seemed to increase in virulence as it flashed across the continent. Thousands of soldiers who were training in camps, on their way to ports of embarkation, aboard troop ships, and arriving at the front in France became ill with the flu. The close quarters and crowded conditions associated with training and transporting military recruits clearly hastened the already rapid spread of the disease. In France, as many soldiers were in the American hospitals because of the flu as because of casualties sustained in combat. In the United States, the draft call was actually canceled in the month of October because the training camp hospitals were so full that they could not hold any more patients.

It has been frequently said that the flu spread among the general population from large to small cities and from urban to rural centers. A civilian case was reported from Boston on September 3, 1918. It seems more probable, however, that the flu escaped from within the army camp in Kansas, and then spread to small towns, villages, and farms in the Midwest. It has also been commonly stated that the flu was relatively mild in the spring, becoming more deadly in August and throughout the autumn. My uncle Robert told me, however, that in Minnesota, "The flu was worst in the spring of the year 1918. At the same time the United States became heavily involved in the war." Almost every family had one or more members who suffered illness, and many families lost loved ones through death. With approximately one-third of all physicians serving in the military, there was a shortage of physicians, and there was an even greater shortage of trained nurses. In addition, the death rate among physicians and nurses was high, especially among those who were twenty to forty years of age. There was also a shortage of supplies, which were needed overseas, and people were urged to make do with what they had.

Edward P. Davis, president of the Volunteer Medical Service Corps, sent a letter to members at the state and county level in which he urged the following: "The Army and Navy are fighting and conquering Germans. We must fight and conquer germs without taking anything away from the Army and Navy. Don't ask the Army and Navy for medical and surgical supplies. Use simple utensils for sterilizing; the simplest kinds of beds and bedding; make your own masks and dressings, and fight for yourselves."

THE FLU IN WABASSO

Cousin Beatrice Fixsen Emmerick was thirteen years old when she came down with the flu. She recovered after being very ill but remembered losing some of her schoolmates. "It just took them," she said, "and it seemed that there was nothing that anybody could do. In the beginning people thought it was like the old-fashioned *la grippe*, but it was much worse, and people became very ill with high fevers. Your father was the only doctor in the community at that time, and he was kept very, very busy."

Uncle Robert told me, "I believe your father never went to bed during that time—it probably shortened his life by five years or so. He hired a driver, George Schueller, and slept while he was being driven from one patient to the next in the sulkey (a horse-drawn buggy). It was impossible to use a car because the roads were so muddy. The driver slept on a cot in the office while waiting to drive the doctor on his calls. It was a terrible time. So many people ran such high fevers and were so very ill."

Arnold J. Bauer reported that the public school was closed in the autumn of 1918 "because of the influenza epidemic becoming so widespread that it was necessary to curb it in this way. Children were not allowed to play together but had to stay on their premises. Occasionally children were found playing together in alleys and these were admonished to refrain from doing so. Sometimes they saw one of the authorities approaching and they dispersed before he could get to them." Mr. Bauer further reported that the celebrating at the end of the First World War was restricted by the influenza epidemic. On Monday, November 11, 1918, "plans were completed for an evening celebration. On account of the influenza it was held in the open on the square at the east end of Main Street."

SYMPTOMS OF THE FLU

The flu's early manifestations were relatively mild. Patients had fevers of 101 to 104 degrees Fahrenheit along with headache, aching muscles, and sometimes drowsiness. Cough, sneezing, and hoarseness were common. The mucous membranes of the nose and throat were usually red, and sometimes hemorrhagic. The conjunctivae (whites of the eyes) were often red. The white blood cell count was normal or low, only increasing if secondary infections occurred. Occasionally there was a transient appearance of albumin in the urine. Most of the early victims recovered after a few days.

The flu became more virulent as it spread. Patients had very high fevers up to 105 degrees, shaking chills, intense prostration, and severe pain in the head, eyes, back, muscles, and joints. The most commonly affected organs were the lungs and the central nervous system. Myocarditis (inflammation of the heart muscles) also occurred, and toxic shock syndrome, unknown at that time but implicated in influenza in recent years, must have been the reason for some of the extremely rapid deaths.

INFLUENZA~PNEUMONIA

The major complication associated with the influenza was pneumonia, and both bronchopneumonia and lobar pneumonia were described. In many instances the rapidly fatal pneumonic process must have been caused by the virus alone. In other cases, there was bacterial as well as viral infection present. When the pneumonia was caused by a secondary bacterial infection, the flu symptoms usually relented for a day or so before worsening. No specific antibiotic was available at that time, of course, for the bacterial pneumonia.

Vividly described in several first-hand accounts was the early, devastating pulmonary edema associated with this severe influenza-pneumonia, which even experienced physicians had never seen before. The illness seemed to come on rapidly, and death could occur within hours of its onset. An army physician whose first name was Roy wrote a touching letter from Camp Devens, Massachusetts, on September 29, 1918, to a physician friend whose first name was Burt about "the most viscious [sic] type of Pneumonia that has ever been seen." He described the clinical course of the disease, as follows: "Two hours after admission they have the Mahogony [sic] spots over the cheek bones, and a few hours later you can begin to see the Cyanosis extending from their ears and spreading all over the face, until it is hard to distinguish the colored men from the white. It is only a matter of a few hours then until death comes, and it is simply a struggle for air until they suffocate. It is horrible."

Isaac Starr was then a medical student at the University of Pennsylvania. He wrote in his recollection of the epidemic in Philadelphia about the "lungs filled with rales, patients short of breath and increasingly cyanotic, gasping for breath, and struggling to clear their airways of a blood-tinged froth that gushed from their nose and mouth. It was a dreadful business."

My parents talked very little about the flu of 1918, but my mother occasionally mentioned that my father could tell immediately from their appearance, that is, their skin color, which patients would not survive. Many of the first-hand accounts of the epidemic described changes that were clearly evidence of severe hypoxia (lack of oxygen). A violaceous, heliotrope cyanosis, changing to maroon and then to a livid bluish-black, was said to characterize hopeless cases. A remarkably vivid description is the one by Carey McCord in his colorful account of how "the purple death," or "the purple plague," affected its victims in Camp Sherman, Chillicothe, Ohio: "To this day no one knows for certain the organism that produced the pneumonia that followed or co-existed with the influenza. Whatever its dreadful nature, that malignant agent produced a purplish, reddish, greyish ashen color of the face—chiefly around the lips, but sometimes over other portions of the body or the entire body. The fluids from the respiratory tract were brilliant pink or red. Hemorrhage was everywhere. Every sheet, towel, pillowcase, gown, whether on a patient, doctor, nurse, or orderly was purplish red. Many who died literally drowned in the bloody waters inside their own bodies."

INFLUENZA-ENCEPHALITIS

Among the most puzzling aspects of the flu, still somewhat controversial today, were the "nervous and mental" components that were often part of the clinical picture. First reported from England, France, and perhaps Austria, these adverse symptoms were difficult to interpret and not immediately recognized as what later came to be called influenza-encephalitis. At first, most physicians thought they were dealing with poliomyelitis or botulism. An editorial in the February 8, 1919, issue of *The Journal of the American Medical Association* labeled it a new disease, encephalitis lethargica, in spite of articles published in the same journal in January and March that described patients who clearly showed the neurotoxic effect of the 1918 influenza virus.

Symptoms of influenza-encephalitis ranged from drowsiness, exhaustion, and prostration to irritability, insomnia, mental aberrations, and delusions. Depression was common and characteristic, usually accompanying the convalescent stages of influenza. Some patients had difficulty concentrating, showed evidence of erratic judgment and inability to reason, and were unable to work. Others were quarrelsome, aggressive, had outbursts of temper, became hysterical, and even displayed active psychotic behavior. McCord, in his description of the purple death, described two soldiers rising from their hospital beds to fight each other in the last few minutes of their lives. The *New York Times* reported that a physician had been killed by a patient who was delirious from influenza.

Sometimes abnormal behaviors coincided with the typical respiratory symptoms of the flu, but more frequently they occurred afterward, following intervals of from a few days to weeks or months or longer.

Well known among such late effects are the tremor and mask-like face that characterize Parkinson's disease. For a time it was thought that a second epidemic of encephalitis lethargica followed or was intertwined with the epidemic of influenza. It is now recognized that influenza-encephalitis, lethargic encephalitis, and post-influenzal Parkinsonism were all caused by the same swine influenza virus and that severe neurological damage from the virus could be immediate and/or could continue through the following years and decades. When I was a medical student, from 1943 through 1946, post-influenzal Parkinsonism was an important differential diagnosis to be considered in evaluating tremors. The incidence of post-encephalitis but not idiopathic (of unknown cause) Parkinson's disease has decreased in recent years.

WHO WAS SPARED?

Another confusing characteristic of the epidemic was that, unlike the usual influenzas of the past, which tended to strike down the very young and the very old, large numbers of vigorous young adults between twenty and forty years of age contracted the flu. At Camp Sherman, Chillicothe, the camp area was overwhelmed by hordes of anxious parents and relatives, and it was feared that these relatives themselves would contract the flu. In fact, this occurred only rarely, and many of the parents slept by their sons' bedsides for a week or longer without becoming ill. The anonymous physician, Roy, reported from Camp Devens to his friend Burt, "We have lost an outrageous number of Nurses and Drs." Dr. McCord at Camp Sherman mentioned the "low incidence of influenza and pneumonia among the older medical officers, who with rare exception remain unaffected." Most of these older people had lived through the 1889-1890 epidemic of "Russian flu" and presumably retained some degree of immunity, even though they may not have been clinically ill at that time.

ETIOLOGY OF THE FLU

There was a great deal of uncertainty in 1918 about the etiology, or cause, of influenza. It was generally accepted that influenza was caused by the Pfeiffer bacillus, a rod-shaped bacterium that could usually be cultured from the sputum of ailing patients. There was also a theory that the causative agent was another organism, which accompanied or rode along with the Pfeiffer bacillus. Pneumococci, hemolytic streptococci, and less commonly, staphylococci, were frequently cultured from the patients' throats, and were thought to cause secondary pneumonia. Attempts to transmit the disease to animals or humans consistently failed, and Victor C. Vaughan, then editor in chief of *The Journal of Laboratory and Clinical Medicine* as well as head of the Army's communicable disease unit, expressed a scientist's viewpoint, "It has not been proven that the Pfeiffer bacillus is or carries the virus of the disease we know as influenza." Not until 1933 did the true viral cause of influenza become established.

TREATMENT OF THE FLU

Because no specific treatment was available (for that matter, specific treatment is not available today), therapy of the flu was symptomatic. Cousin Beatrice Emmerick described what she knew of my father's efforts. "He would do whatever he could, even packing patients in ice to try to bring down the fevers, but there was nothing, really, that anyone was able to do." Uncle Robert Daub said, "I believe Dr. Brey used quinine and perhaps morphine to treat the patients—that's all there was."

The Therapeutics section of the October 5, 1918, *Journal of the American Medical Association* recommended acetylsalicylic acid (aspirin) and phenacetin (the ethyl ether of acetaminophen) for pain, as well as fluids and bed rest. No mention was made of aspirin for relief of fever. Chilling was to be avoided to prevent complications. When pneumonia supervened, warm packs were considered useful, combined with cold applications to the head. The "toxemia" of pneumonia could be combated by giving fluids by mouth, proctoclysis (by rectum), or hypodermoclysis (under the skin). No mention was made of the intravenous route; that method of administering fluids had not yet been perfected.

Prostration was to be combated with stimulants such as caffeine, sodium benzoate, digitalis, strophanthus, and camphorated oil. Oxygen was advised for marked cyanosis. Epinephrin [sic] (adrenaline) was suggested for vasomotor depression. Morphin [sic] and large doses of atropin [sic] were recommended for the massive flood of fluid into the lungs and bronchi that often marked the final stages of pneumonia.

In desperation, physicians sometimes reverted to the "heroic measures" that had fallen into disrepute during the preceding century. The *Journal of the American Medical Association* even recommended, for secondary pneumonia, purging with large doses of magnesium citrate salts or calomel and stated that in severe cases "venesection (bleeding) may prove extremely valuable." For patients with pneumonia, it further suggested injecting the citrated blood of a convalescent person into the muscles of the patient in order to provide specific antibodies. The blood should test negative for syphilis, of course, but this procedure was otherwise "devoid of any harmful effects."

PREVENTION OF THE FLU

Preventive measures did not seem to be particularly effective, although there was a great deal known by then about how to avoid contracting contagious diseases. Cousin Beatrice Emmerick said, "I remember that we (children) were quarantined. We didn't go to school and we weren't to play together, but the flu spread anyway to so many people—and not only the elderly."

Influenza spread through respiratory secretions contained in airborn droplets and by hand-to-mouth transfer from contaminated objects and surfaces. Edward P. Davis advised the members of the Volunteer Medical Service Corps to "instruct families under their care to guard against the epidemic by:

- Thorough cleanliness of houses, premises, clothing, utensils, and personal cleanliness.
- Avoid stirring up dust.

- Wash; scrub; flush; sprinkle; and use soap and water thoroughly.

- Gargle and spray the nose and throat with an alkaline antiseptic frequently.

- Urge the importance of fresh air and the avoidance of chill and overheat.

- Give no medicine and use no treatment which may depress the vital forces, especially the heart of the patient.

Sometimes the efforts aimed toward prevention seemed to be merely frantic and without merit. For example, quarantine, which included closing schools, theaters, saloons, and churches, and forbidding public burials, was not especially effective. Many countries attempted to restrict ships from using their ports in the hope of preventing the spread of the flu. These efforts were almost always useless, usually because the embargo was too late. However, the South Sea Islands of Samoa experienced sharply different results in their efforts to prevent infection. In Western Samoa, the flu was introduced by a ship from New Zealand, while in American Samoa, only seventy kilometers away, strict quarantine was effective in preventing the flu from reaching the island.

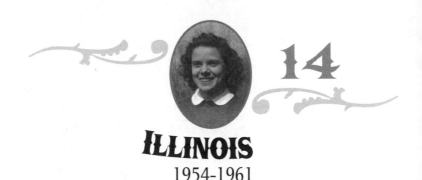

ILLINOIS
1954-1961

e moved to the Chicago area in 1954 for Fran's first job when he became an assistant professor at Northwestern University. His office was in the Veterans' Administration Research Hospital in Chicago. We moved to a small house, our first, in Arlington Heights, and our son, Rick, started kindergarten. Our daughter Carol had been delivered at Midway Hospital in St. Paul on February 13, 1953, by Dr. Jane Hodgson, and she was approximately 18 months old at the time of our move. Carol was a very active child who quickly learned to walk and talk. In fact, she was a very talkative little girl. Her most outstanding characteristic, which developed at a very early age, was her capacity for great sympathy and empathy with people and animals.

A UNIQUE EXPERIENCE

One of our first efforts was to sit for the Illinois state medical board examination so that we could be licensed to practice medicine in Illinois. Fran and I obtained Minnesota licenses by examination in 1947, immediately after completing our internships, and we retained those licenses throughout our active careers. Minnesota reciprocated with most states, so that obtaining a new license in another state was usually only a formality—subsequent licenses in Oklahoma, Michigan, the District of Columbia, and Virginia were all obtained through reciprocity.

Illinois did not reciprocate, however, and therefore we were required to take their state board examination.

We had taken many examinations throughout the years, but this one was a truly unique, even shocking, experience. The examination took place in a large auditorium filled with foreigners, most of them men, and most of them not fluent in English. This was the post-WWII period, and these were persons who were trying to gain entry to the United States. It was bedlam. There was a great deal of noise and moving about. The monitors were almost frantic, trying to prevent cheating, but they could not prevent the men from taking frequent trips to the restrooms. The man who was sitting immediately behind me kept hissing in my ear, "Schick test! What is a Schick test?" (A Schick test is a skin test, no longer in standard use, that determines whether an individual is immune to diphtheria.) We met only one U.S. trained physician; an obstetrician, he told us the answer to one of the examination questions after the examination was over. An infant delivered by Caesarian section must be extracted in less than three minutes, he said, in order to insure that the baby has adequate oxygen. We passed the examination but heard later that very few of the other examinees had passed.

Too Busy

This was the aftermath of WWII, and a time when a great many young men (and some women) who had returned from service were marrying, having children, and looking for their first homes. A number of affordable housing developments were being built in our area, most notably an extremely large one called Rolling Meadows. The local population of young people with young families was burgeoning. The population of Chicago was shifting to the western suburbs, but the professionals needed to care for them were slower to follow this shift. As a result, there was a shortage of physicians, and the ones who were there were overburdened. I began practicing general pediatrics alone but was soon overwhelmed by the demand for my services and by being constantly on call.

COLLEAGUES

After a year of going it alone, I joined Elfriede "Fee" Horst in her general pediatric practice in Des Plaines, and a few years later we recruited Patricia "Pat" Conard to become the third partner in the practice. All three of us had husbands and young children; Fee had a boy and a girl, and Pat had four girls. Being on call every third night gave us time to be with our families, and working only every third night seemed almost like being on vacation. When one of us was away, it was necessary to be on call every second night, and when two were away, one person was left to work every day and every night. Fortunately the latter situation was extremely rare. The three of us got along well because we shared similar interests and obligations, especially our concerns about raising our children. Fee's experience and good medical judgment, along with Pat's recent training and intelligence made both of them outstanding persons to be associated with. We became firm friends and supported each other through various personal and domestic crises with advice and sympathy.

We referred patients to various specialists in the area; all of them were competent, gave good service to the children and their parents, and reported back to us concerning their findings. Several of them had certain quirks, however, that we needed to consider before sending patients to them. One was a nationally known neurologist who had a well-deserved reputation as one of the very best in his field. He had, however, a very grumpy personality, and we had to warn the families that he was "cranky, but if you can overlook that, he will give you the correct diagnosis for your child." They would invariably inform us when they came back later that he "wasn't so bad after all." Another was a neurosurgeon who frequently refused to talk to families after a surgical procedure. Many of his little patients had serious diseases such as hydrocephalus (water on the brain) or a brain tumor. He was an extremely sensitive individual and was sometimes reported to be crying in the dressing room after an operation. We, then, would talk to the families, explaining the surgical results and letting them know that their surgeon was so sorry about the outcome that he couldn't face them. They would always express sympathy for him and say that they understood. Still another was an ENT (ear, nose, and throat) specialist who did not believe in analgesics (pain relievers). We would have the family bring the child to our office on their way home from an ENT visit, and we would administer an injection of Demerol (a potent pain reliever) or prescribe a medication that could be taken by mouth.

NEIGHBORS

Our little house in Arlington Heights was located in a blue-collar neighborhood. We were quite happy with the house and had pleasant neighbors on either side of us. The rest of the neighbors, however, disliked me—I think they resented my having household help and an automobile. Their attitude became a problem because they ostracized our children and frightened our housekeeper, Mattie. However, they didn't hesitate to call me, especially at night if they had a medical problem with a child. I discussed this with my mother, who said, "I don't think you have any alternative but to move." We did move, to Mount Prospect, a more affluent neighborhood, and there were no more such problems. I have talked to other women physicians who reported being similarly resented and ostracized while living in a blue-collar neighborhood.

CALLED BACK INTO SERVICE

We were disappointed, but not surprised, when Fran was called back into the Army after the Korean War. It didn't seem quite fair, since we now had two children, and for the first time we were both gainfully employed. Fran had no choice, however, but to serve his country. He had been discharged from his assignment in Panama, because of an old eye problem, before his two years of payback to the Army was completed, and he was therefore eligible for re-induction to serve two full years. Fortunately, he was assigned for most of that time to a laboratory in Fort Knox and was able to come home by train every Friday night and stay until Sunday evening. On Monday through Thursday nights he moonlighted at Norton Memorial Infirmary in Louisville, Kentucky. It's a bit difficult to know when he slept, but I think he did his sleeping on the train, coming and going.

When he was given an honorable discharge after two years of service, he had served 14 years in the Army, either on active duty or in the reserves. He could have remained in the military reserve following discharge, and in six years he would have been eligible for a 20 year pension. Because we were worried that he might be conscripted again, however, we both agreed that he should, and he did, accept a final discharge at that time.

ALICE

Our third child, Alice, was born after Fran was discharged from his third tour of duty in the Army. She was delivered at Resurrection Hospital in Chicago by Fee's husband, Arthur Levan. We were surprised and extremely upset to learn that we had a black-and-blue baby. Interestingly, neither the obstetric nor the newborn nursery staff noticed that our newborn infant was covered with bruises from her head to her feet. The problem was not recognized until my partner, Fee, came in the next morning to carry out a routine newborn checkup and immediately started investigating. Alice had a most unusual group of problems, thrombocytopenia (a low platelet count) complicated by hemolytic anemia. We were terrified that she would bleed into her brain because of the bleeding problem, but fortunately that did not happen. The hemolytic anemia, which developed later, was severe enough to require a blood transfusion every five days. (The anemia was due to hemolysis of the red blood cells, that is, the red cells breaking down faster than they can be replaced by the body.) We were so worried by this time that we simply took each day as it came and tried not to think about what else could happen.

Alice was cared for in Bobs Roberts Hospital for Children at the University of Chicago by Dr. Mila Pierce. Dr. Pierce was a pediatric hematologist/oncologist, one of the early pioneers in the treatment of childhood leukemia, and a very gracious lady. We came to recognize her as a savvy physician and a kind person. No one ever made an official diagnosis of Alice's problem, but she responded to an exchange transfusion, multiple platelet and red cell transfusions, and a course of prednisone treatment. Fran had recently been discharged from the Army, we had very little money, we were away from the help and support of our extended family, and we needed to find blood donors for our baby. My mother communicated this to my family, and some of my family members in Minnesota gave blood to the Red Cross, which was credited to our account in Chicago. By six months of age Alice had improved so that she no longer needed blood transfusions, and the prednisone was discontinued. We still owed the blood bank, however, and we decided that the right thing would be to replace the blood rather than to give them money for what we owed. Fran eventually paid back all of the blood owed to the blood bank by donating his own blood every three to six months over a period of several years until the debt was paid. In later years I came to believe, after discussing the problem with Dr. Wolf Zuelzer, that Alice must have had a viral infection, transmitted from mother to infant.

CHILD CARE

As it is for all families in which both parents work outside the home, child care was a problem [Figure 34]. We advertised and hired our first nanny, Mrs. Maley, an older woman whom we liked very much. She developed a tremor, however, and it became clear that she could not safely lift Carol, who was close to 24 months old at the time. We advertised and found Mattie, who came out from the inner city of Chicago on Monday mornings and stayed until Friday night. She began showing up later and later on Monday mornings, so we advertised again for help. Mrs. Fahey was with us for a short time, but she, too, was not dependable. Eventually Mrs. Isabella Leslie, a lovely red-haired Scottish woman straight from Scotland, responded to our ad and became the answer to

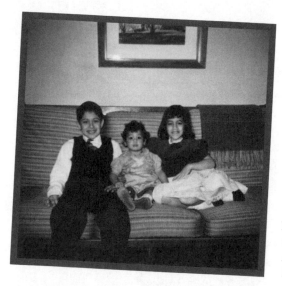

Fig. 34: *Rick, age 9 ½ years, Carol, age 6 ½ years, and Alice, age 1 ½ years, in Mount Prospect, Illinois, 1959.*

our prayers. I was pregnant with Alice when she first came to work for us, and she remained with us until Alice was eight years old, even moving with us to Oklahoma. "Nana" was what she asked the children to call her. She shared our home and was with us through our sorrows and (mostly) joys. It is difficult to adequately express how much we all benefited from her help and support during those important years when our children were growing up.

MOVE TO OKLAHOMA

Fran received an offer from the University of Oklahoma that he could not refuse. From being an assistant professor at Northwestern University, he bypassed the associate professor level and became a full professor and chairman of the Department of Physiology at the University of Oklahoma Medical School. I was sorry to lose the emotional support of my two partners when the time came for Fran and me to move our family to Oklahoma, but we remained friends and kept in touch. Unfortunately, Fee died several years after I left Illinois, leaving her husband and her children Katie and Peter to mourn. Pat remains in good health; we keep in touch and we see her and her husband, Dr. Paul Birk, on occasion.

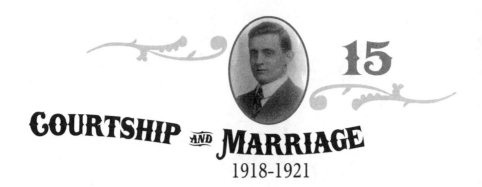

COURTSHIP and MARRIAGE
1918-1921

P ublic health began to come into its own around the turn of the century, and by then most states and large cities had health departments. The Hygiene Laboratory in Washington, D.C., which was opened in 1901, became the National Institutes of Health in 1930. The United States Public Health service was established in 1912. It was successful in its efforts to eliminate yellow fever, hookworm, and pellagra. In 1918 it greatly increased the scope of its operations with a much larger budget. This was, in part, in response to the need for control of venereal diseases, which had greatly increased in prevalence, especially among the military personnel who were involved in the First World War. In 1921 Canadian researchers Banting and Best isolated insulin, and patients with diabetes mellitis were given an opportunity to lead a more normal life.

Courtship in those days was not hurried. The romantic interest between my father and mother was evidently awakened during the flu epidemic of 1918, although they surely must have known each other, or at least of each other, before then. After the epidemic was over, he asked her to stay on as his office nurse, and she continued to live at home while working for him [Figure 35].

People tended to entertain themselves, visiting with relatives or friends, playing card games, going on picnics, and attending church

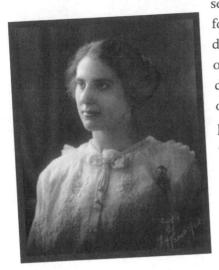

Fig. 35: *Elizabeth Katherine Daub, circa 1920.*

services and church socials. The young folks danced and played cards but drinking and smoking were not part of their lives. My parents did not drink alcohol, smoke, use illicit drugs, or gamble. My father may have accompanied my mother and her family to church on occasion (although he was never very strong on church attendance while I was growing up). The Daub family had been involved in the building of St. Anne's Roman Catholic Church in Wabasso, even contributing one of the stained glass windows, and they were regular church goers.

Music was an important leisure activity. There was a piano in the Daub home, and my mother's sister Anne was the pianist. Aunt Anne's sheet music for a number of the lovely popular songs of the time remained for many years in the piano bench in the parlor of their farm home. Among her individual pieces of sheet music were "Beautiful Ohio," "The Missouri Waltz," "Silver Bell," and "Tuck Me to Sleep in My Old 'Tucky Home." Other well liked songs such as "Home, Sweet Home," "My Darling Nelly Gray," and those of Stephen C. Foster were included in *The Golden Book of Favorite Songs*. My mother was especially fond of "She'll Be Comin' Round the Mountain." Perhaps the most beloved songs of all were the hauntingly beautiful songs of the Civil War that had been revived because of the ongoing First World War, "Battle Hymn of the Republic," "The Vacant Chair," "Tramp, Tramp, Tramp," "Tenting on the Old Camp Ground," "Just Before the Battle, Mother," "When Johnny Comes Marching Home," and a new one that had been written for the current war, "Keep the Home Fires Burning." When I was a small child, I thought "The Vacant Chair" had been written about my Uncle Joe because of the line about "his mild blue eyes."

All of the members of the Daub family had eyes of various shades of blue. My mother's older brother Joseph, the only relative that I know of who served in the military during the First World War, had such faded blue eyes. He, unlike the soldier in the song, survived and came safely home after the war.

Cousin Beatrice Fixsen Emmerick told this anecdote about my parents' courtship: "I remember once when your Aunt Helen and I were high school kids, and I was out at your Grandfather Daub's farm visiting Helen. In the evening the men were sitting around the table talking, as men do, when Dr. Brey came. Your mother ran upstairs. She had to fix her hair, but she fussed around with it and did a hundred other things. Her eyes were shining and she looked excited, but she kept finding excuses why she couldn't go down. Her sisters Anne and Therese were up there with her.

"Finally Anne, in her practical, matter of fact manner said to Elizabeth, 'I don't see why you don't go down. You look all right. He came to see you.'

"And Therese echoed, with a smile, 'I don't know why you don't go down.'

"Here were the men downstairs around the table, your Grandfather Daub and John and Louie and Joe and Robert and Doc, all sitting and talking—talking about crops, business, the times, financial things, and having a good time. And here was your mother, upstairs, wanting to come down but a little bashful. I really don't know how they ever got together, but they evidently did! She must have come down eventually, of course, but your Grandmother Daub packed Helen and me off to bed before that happened.

"In the meantime, Helen and I had a wonderful time, running back and forth, watching what was going on upstairs and downstairs, and giggling and enjoying ourselves like the teenagers we were."

Beatrice also said, "I remember when Elizabeth came to be his nurse; that's when they started going together. And when they were quite serious, there was some kind of rift—I don't know just what it was all about—but Elizabeth said, 'It's all over, all over.' Of course it wasn't. I don't remember their wedding; I was probably away at school at the time."

Two letters have been preserved, both written by my father in November, 1920, to Miss Elizabeth Daub in care of Mercy Hospital, Devil's Lake, North Dakota, where my mother's sister Clara was ill. Clara, who was training to be a nurse, had typhoid fever, and my mother had gone there to be with her. Clara never finished her training. My father and mother must have been thinking about marrying each other (they were married a year later); his letters seem to express concern about his ability to support a family. In the first letter he wrote:

Tuesday Morning
Postmarked Nov 2, 1920
Dearest Elizabeth;

I got your letter Saturday and see Clara is still pretty sick, also saw Henry since he came home and hoped he would be able to report a big improvement, but he also told me that there isn't much. Hope she is by the next time I hear from you.

You won't need to worry about getting work when you get back. That is, to earn money. I am earning plenty for us to get along if I just stick to the job. It's sometimes a little hard for me to collect it after I have earned it.

I was real busy Sunday and yesterday. We had a little snow Sunday PM and rain yesterday. There is a little snow on the ground now, but the sun is out and I guess it will be gone at noon.

With best wishes and hopes that everything will soon be well where you are. I close with

Love,
Frank

The Henry he referred to in the above letter was Henry Goblirsch, who later married Clara and became my uncle by marriage. In the second letter he again mentioned his work:

Wabasso, Minn
11/11/20
Postmarked Nov 12
Dearest Elizabeth:

Received your letter and am glad Clara is better and hope she is out of danger now (at this writing).

What you mention about yourself I think will gradually get better and after a while subside completely.

I am still doing good business. It seems all I need to do is stick close to the job and I always have work.

I put the net in Sunday. It rained Monday so I didn't need to take it out, Louie took [it] out and had about 10 big pickerel, he also got a couple of ducks. I haven't hunted nor fished at all yet. Yesterday and today everything froze over.

Excuse my short letters. Must close with best wishes to both of you.

With love,
Frank

My parents were married on Thanksgiving Day, November 24, 1921, in the church of St. Anne in Wabasso, with my mother's sister Therese and her brother Joseph as their attendants.

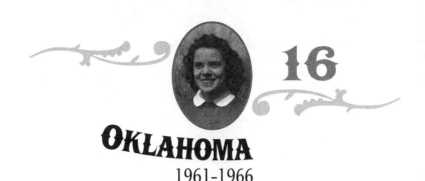

OKLAHOMA
1961–1966

Our five years in Oklahoma were good years for our family. As we traveled south to our new home in Oklahoma City, we looked rather doubtfully at the terrain, at the short trees and the yellow ochre and burnt sienna colors of the landscape, so different from the tall trees and the greens and blues of Minnesota and Illinois. However, we came to appreciate the beauty of the Oklahoma terrain. We also appreciated the people, who were open and friendly. At one of my first encounters in a convenience store, where we stopped on our way, a man called me "Honey." I thought to myself, I am going to like this state! I was told later that in the South and Southwest women are called "Honey" and men are called "Son." Nana came with us, and our children, who were then eleven, eight, and three years old, did well in Oklahoma.

When Fran joined the University of Oklahoma Medical School, he left his position as an assistant professor at Northwestern University, bypassed the associate professor level, and became full professor and chair of the Department of Physiology in the University of Oklahoma Medical School. Although the University's main campus is in Norman, the medical school is located in Oklahoma City, and we lived in a large, old house, within walking distance of the school and hospital.

HOME AND CHILDREN

The pleasant neighborhood we lived in had an oil field beneath it, and an oil pump was located one block west of our house. Some of our neighbors were receiving small yearly payments for the oil that presumably came from beneath their property. We did not receive such payments because the "mineral rights" to our property had been sold to an oil company when the house changed hands previously. Our house, which was only a few blocks north of the medical school, was only a few blocks south of the state capitol building. Another oil pump, located next to the capitol, pumped oil from under the complex of state buildings. We, of course, forbid our children to go near any of the oil pumps.

Rick and Carol, who were very active children, were at first allowed to run all over the neighborhood, except for the oil fields. They began bringing home autographed photographs of the various legislators, however, and we learned that they were visiting the legislators' offices in the state buildings. Their favorite photo (and ours) was of Cowboy Pink Williams, a well-known state politician whose colorful name gave him instant recognition throughout Oklahoma. We, of course, also forbid them to go into the state capitol buildings, but we were never quite sure that they obeyed any of our instructions.

Alice developed from a baby to a preschooler and school child, a bright-eyed little girl who observed everything that went on. She could talk but never seemed to have much to say. We were amazed when her teacher told us after she started kindergarten that she was a very good pupil.

OKLAHOMA NATIVE AMERICANS

We learned a lot about Southwestern history. There are many Native American tribes in Oklahoma, many having been banished from other states. Oklahoma does not have reservations, but, rather, Indian-owned lands, and the Native Americans mix freely among the population. A large proportion of Oklahomans claim some Indian ancestry, and some are wealthy, mostly from oil money. Your legislator, your physician, your hairdresser, the person who assists you in the drug store, any of these individuals is likely to be a Native American. Our next door neighbors were a charming married couple who were both of partial Indian ancestry and whose son, a graduate of West Point and an artist, sculpted a bust of our son. One of my teachers, later a friend and colleague, at the University of Oklahoma Medical School was Dr. James Hampton, a member of the Choctaw tribe, who became the first Native American oncologist in the United States.

AN ACADEMIC CAREER

Before we left Illinois, I heard from Dr. Harris D. "Pete" Riley, who chaired the Department of Pediatrics in the University of Oklahoma Medical School, offering me a position in his department. I gladly accepted the offer, and thus began my career in academic medicine. The department needed a pediatric hematologist/oncologist because the previous staff member who sub-specialized in the diseases of blood and cancer in children had recently resigned and moved away. The department had a grant from the National Institutes of Health, which had been awarded to a principal investigator for clinical research on childhood cancer, and the department needed a principal investigator for the grant. So I became a pediatric hematologist/oncologist. Dr. Riley was at all times a sympathetic and supportive chair. Our family lived close to his and our families became friends, especially our Alice and their little daughter Margaret, who were the same age and who enjoyed some good times together.

PEDIATRIC HEMATOLOGY/ONCOLOGY

I knew very little about blood diseases and cancer in children, so an arrangement was made for me to work under the supervision of Dr. Robert Bird, who was the director of hematology and oncology in the Department of Medicine. Specialists in internal medicine had to take separate board examinations to become subspecialists in medical hematology and medical oncology. For pediatricians, such as myself, pediatric hematology/oncology was combined and required a single board examination. I received advice and counsel from Dr. Bird and the other members of his group. As a fellow in hematology/oncology and, at the same time, an instructor in pediatrics, I regularly went on hospital rounds with my medical colleagues and customarily turned to them for help when I needed consultation. My close collaboration with the medical hematologists and oncologists in Oklahoma formed the pattern for how I would continue to function when I worked in other institutions because I was usually the only pediatrician who was doing hematology/oncology. In addition to Dr. Bird, other members of the medical hematology and oncology team included Dick Marshall and Jim Hampton. When I first knew Jim he was a medical hematologist, subspecializing in blood clotting disorders, and I thought of him as a quiet person, almost shy, but extremely intelligent and competent. He later concentrated on oncology and became director of the cancer center in Oklahoma City, the first Native American oncologist and the first Native American director of a cancer center.

LEAVING OKLAHOMA

We left Oklahoma in 1966 with great reluctance. Our five years there were happy ones. We made good friends, our children thrived, and Fran and I enjoyed our work at the University of Oklahoma Medical School. The problem was that at that time the state did not adequately fund its schools of higher education, and Fran had been supporting his physiology department with grant funds for five years. Now the federal sources of grant funds were becoming less easy to obtain. He decided to accept a position as chair of physiology at Michigan State University, which was starting a new medical school. There were a number of open positions at MSU, so that he was able to offer positions to people on his Oklahoma staff who would otherwise soon lose their jobs and paychecks. A number of them accepted and moved with us to Michigan.

Among those who moved with us to Michigan were Booker T. Swindall, who had worked with Fran in Chicago, Joe and Loretta Dabney, and Jerry and Doris Scott. By this time Nana felt that she had brought Alice through the important infant and early childhood years, and she decided not to go with us. Nana died several years later in retirement in Canada, at the home of one of her daughters.

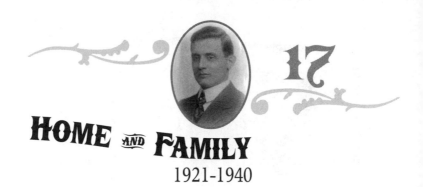

HOME AND FAMILY
1921-1940

he name "vitamine" was invented in 1912, around the time that preventive medicine was beginning to be concerned with nutritional disorders. Elmer V. McCollum, working at the University of Wisconsin, discovered vitamin A in 1913 and vitamin D in 1922 by feeding rats on selective diets. It was established by 1915 that deficiency of vitamin B caused pellagra, but it was not known until 1937 that pellagra responded to niacin (nicotinic acid), one of the B vitamins. The role of citrus fruits in preventing and curing scurvy had been known for some time, since before 1800; how best to preserve vitamin C in food preparation now became the focus of attention. The discovery of ultra violet as an antirachitic agent in 1922 and the identification of ergosterol as provitamin C in 1927 were followed by a remarkable reduction in the number of cases of rickets. Iodized salt was marketed in grocery stores after a nutritional deficiency of iodine was shown to be a common cause of goiter, especially among people who lived in the Great Lakes region.

As a newly wed couple, my parents moved into the house we continued to occupy throughout the time the family lived in Wabasso [Figure 36]. My sister Ann Catherine (Ann) was born on November 22, 1922, and the rest of us followed closely: Theresa Eileen (Terry) on February 27, 1924;

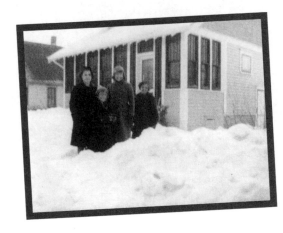

FIG. 36: *Photograph (left to right) of Theresa, Justine, Ann, and Virginia in front of the Brey home, circa 1934.*

Alois John (Al) on April 28, 1925; Virginia Carroll (Ginger) on July 18, 1926; Paul Daub on December 30, 1927; and Justine Elizabeth (Teeny) on February 11, 1929. We grew up in a child-centered home. It always seemed to me that my father thought the most wonderful thing that had ever happened to him was to have a family of six children. He and my mother were devoted parents, and they gave a good deal of thought to what was best for us. If they were overprotective at times, we understood that it was because they loved us.

The house, with its three bedrooms, one shared by my parents, the second by my brothers, and the third by us four girls, soon became too small for our family. The front porch was enclosed, giving us extra play room on rainy days, and an extension was built on to the back of our three-bedroom house, adding a kitchen/family room on the first floor and a sleeping porch on the second. My three sisters and I used the bedroom as a dressing room and slept in two double beds in the unheated sleeping porch. It was sometimes quite cold during those Minnesota winters, but we had lots of warm blankets, and, anyway, wasn't fresh air known to be good for everyone? For example, at that time fresh air was considered to be extremely significant in the treatment of tuberculosis.

As busy as he was with his growing family and his medical practice, my father never failed in his attention to his and my mother's parents and siblings, as well as their siblings' spouses and children. We always celebrated Christmas with my mother's family, and also New Year's, which was Grandma Daub's birthday. We celebrated the Fourth of July with Grandma Brey because her birthday fell on that date [Figures 37 and 38]. Uncle Anton Brey was always in charge of the fireworks on the Fourth. My father placed special emphasis upon the area of child safety, and because of his awareness, none of us was allowed near the fireworks.

He continued to find time for a remarkable number of other interests. Most important was his dedication to education, for the children in the community in general and for his own children in particular. He continued to enjoy hunting in the local fields. Other interests included gardening, farming, and politics.

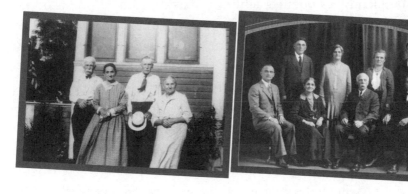

(From Left To Right)
Fig. 37: *All four grandparents together at a Fourth of July celebration, circa 1936, photograph (left to right) of Grandpa Brey, Grandma Brey, Grandpa Daub, and Grandma Daub.*

Fig. 38: *Photograph of the Brey family, probably taken at the parents' golden wedding, circa 1931. Front row, seated, from left, Joseph Brey, Anna Altmann Brey, Alois Brey, and Louie Brey. Back row, standing, from left, Anton Brey, Mary Brey Gliesner, Theresa Brey Goblirsch, and Frank W. Brey.*

CHILDREN'S EDUCATION

My father served as a member of the Wabasso School Board from 1929 to 1940 and was its president from 1932 to 1940. He took a deep interest in what we children were learning in school. He often questioned us about what was going on at school, and he made sure that we all did our homework. He had a special love for the English language, and he enjoyed discussing with us various points of grammar and English usage. He felt that it was very important for us to learn to speak correctly. He and my mother had been brought up in German-speaking homes, in which the children were not exposed to English until they started school, and he believed that this had placed him at a disadvantage. Therefore, although our parents were fluent in German, the only German we ever heard spoken in our home was an occasional word or phrase spoken to each other when they wished to have a private conversation.

Before I started the first grade (the Wabasso school system did not have a kindergarten for Ann and me, but one was started the next year and consequently my younger siblings, starting with Al, went to kindergarten), my father was already planning to send the whole lot of us to college. We would all attend the University of Minnesota, he said, because he could not afford to send six children to private colleges. Tuition at the state university would be low, and our primary expenses would be for room, board, and textbooks. In order to minimize costs, he and my mother would purchase a house near the university, and my mother would live there and manage the household during the school year while he continued his medical practice in Wabasso. There would, of course, be gossip in the village that my parents had separated, but he and my mother felt that this could be tolerated because of the advantage to be derived from the arrangement.

ANN

The birth of their first child was very exciting for my parents, who were older parents by the standards of the day. Figure 39 shows Ann as an infant, being held in Aunt Anne Daub's arms in front of our house. In the background is the Model T Ford automobile owned by my father and used to make house calls. Figure 40 shows Ann, almost three years old with me, 18 months old. Ann had a series of difficult ear infections, starting in early infancy, and with no antibiotic therapy available, a painful myringotomy (an incision of the ear drum to allow pus to drain from the middle ear) was required on occasion. These procedures, which were carried out by my father and needed to be done at the optimal time, before the ear drum ruptured from pressure, must have been almost as painful to him. They accomplished their purpose because she never developed mastoiditis (an infection of the mastoid bone, located behind the ear, a common complication of ear infections before antibiotics were available) and her hearing remained intact (hearing loss was another common complication of ear infections).

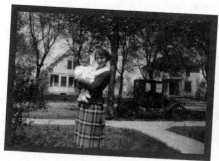 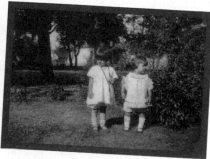

(From Left To Right)
Fig. 39: *Photograph of Anne Daub holding Ann Brey as an infant, in front of the Brey home, in the Spring of 1923. Dr. Brey's Model T automobile stands in the street on the right.*

Fig. 40: *Photograph of Ann and Theresa in front of the Brey home, August 30, 1925.*

Ann's interests were chiefly domestic ones, such as cooking, sewing, canning, decorating, and crafts, and she enjoyed helping our mother organize the household. She was able to wallpaper a room, sew a quilt, and make root beer in the basement without being taught by anyone— our mother never did any of those things. The bottles of root beer tended to pop their corks at inconvenient times, sometimes in the middle of the night. The root beer that survived, however, was delicious.

THERESA

My father was my role model, and my esteem for the work he did was the reason why I chose medicine for my profession. When I was five years old, I first said that I wanted to be a doctor when I grew up. By that time I had rejected both of my mother's occupations: nursing, which she dearly loved and hoped to return to some day (she did, after my father died), and housekeeping, which she despised (as distinguished from homemaking, which she enjoyed, as I do). My mother felt that I should be discouraged from considering medicine as a profession because there were then very few women physicians. My father, on the other hand, felt sure that women would be better accepted by the time I would be ready for medical school, and he counseled my mother not to discourage me. He sometimes talked about the women students he had known when he was a medical student. "We called them 'hens'," he said, "'hen medics'."

Interestingly, a paper published in the *Journal of the American Medical Association* in 1985 reported that among women physicians, the majority had physicians for fathers and considered their fathers to have been the most important factor influencing their choice of career. As it turned out, six of 104 students in my 1943 entering medical school class at the University of Minnesota were women. We were better accepted than the women students of my father's day—nobody called us "hen medics"—but not nearly as well as young women are accepted as medical students today.

ALOIS

My brother Al, named Alois after Grandpa Brey, was teased at school for having a "girl's" name, but the teasing didn't bother him unduly. He was the kind of well-behaved boy who "never put a foot wrong." Figure 41 shows him at three years of age with my mother and several siblings in a wooden sleigh that remained throughout the summers in the alley behind our house. In winter, when the snow was too deep for his Model T to get through, my father sometimes used the sleigh, drawn by a pair of horses, for making house calls. At other times, he rode horseback or walked. I don't believe he especially enjoyed riding horses, but, having been brought up on a farm, he certainly knew how. Al spent several summers with Uncle Anton Brey's family on the Brey family farm. Grandfather Brey had retired by that time, and Anton was now running the "home place." This influence was no doubt part of the reason for my brother's interest in agriculture.

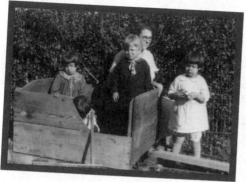

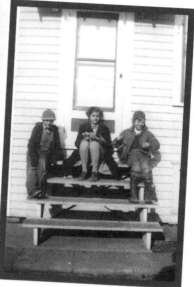

(From Left To Right)
Fig. 41: *Photograph of Virginia, age two, Alois, age three, mother, Theresa, age four, and Ann (looking downward) , age five, in the alley behind the Brey home, circa 1928. Three of the children are sitting in the sleigh used by Dr. Brey to make house calls in winter when the snow was deep.*

Fig. 42: *Photograph of David Goblirsch, Virginia, and Paul, sitting on the back steps of the Brey home, circa 1932.*

Ⅴ︁IRGINIA

Ginger [Figure 42] talked very little, and when she began dropping things at about three years of age, it was not immediately obvious that she had weakness of both hands. My parents took her to the Mayo Clinic for yearly consultations, and it was at first suspected that she had an unusual form of progressive muscular dystrophy. In fact, my father's medical record at the Mayo Clinic, when he was seen there for his final illness in 1939-1940, carries the incorrect notation that one of his children had muscular dystrophy. After being followed for a number of years, it became clear that her status was not worsening, but improving.

She most probably had had a "missed" case of infantile paralysis, that is, one that was undiagnosed in its acute phase. Poliomyelitis is more likely to affect the lower than the upper extremities, that is, the legs and thighs rather than the hands and arms. Furthermore, a symmetrical pattern affecting nerves and muscles on both sides, especially of the hands, had either not yet been described or was not commonly known. Because the early symptoms of polio are similar to those of the common cold, it would be easy to miss the diagnosis, especially in such an uncomplaining child. The mild, almost imperceptible weakness that persisted (for example, she was unable to lift a bowling ball) did not deter Ginger from becoming a nurse when she grew up.

PAUL

Protective as my parents were, they considered Wabasso and its environs to be safe for children, and we were allowed to wander freely through the village and to hike out into the surrounding farms. Paul and our cousin David Goblirsch, Aunt Clara and Uncle Henry's son, were the same age and close friends. Their activities were a recurring source of mixed concern, especially to my father with his worry about child safety, and amusement to both sets of parents, even though they never knew about many of their exploits—for example, the times they went swimming without supervision.

Nor did their parents know that the boys spent a great deal of time hanging around the railroad. They had been forbidden to go there because of the danger from climbing around the trains, and also because it was possible to fall into a loaded boxcar and be unable to get out. People had been known to smother in the grain before help could come. Further, there was no assurance that the homeless men who hung around the depot were not dangerous. The boys left pennies on the railroad tracks and picked up the flattened pennies after the trains had passed over them. They threw rocks and broke the blue glass insulators that hung above the yardarms. They were in and out of boxcars, usually but not always empty ones, and sometimes the trains began to move before they climbed out. Fortunately, they came to no harm.

Their parents did learn of some of their enterprises. One evening when Paul returned home to say that he and David had been boating on Daub's Lake, my mother asked, "Where did you find a boat?" Said Paul, "We found one chained to a tree. We couldn't break the padlock, but the tree was small, so we just chopped the tree down and went off with the boat!" My mother could hardly wait until my father came home that night to tell him about it. They laughed about it together, after we children were in bed, supposedly asleep, and somehow the subject of punishment never came up.

One Sunday afternoon the boys were banished from a bazaar at St. Anne's Church after they had been caught dropping brown paper bags full of water from a second story window on people below. They hiked out into the countryside; there they decided to console themselves with a marshmallow roast. The fire from their bonfire spread to a nearby haystack, and in turn to a field of dried cornstalks. The church bazaar broke up when the congregation heard the local fire engine clanging its bell on the way toward the fire, with flames and smoke easily visible from the church. As usual, the idea of punishment somehow became lost in the confusion.

The boys' most notable accomplishment was when they chopped down the bandstand. The bandstand was a gazebo-like, white-painted, wooden construction, just large enough to contain the band members. It was placed in the center of the village park for concerts, but when not in use, it was transported to a vacant lot and left there until needed for the next concert. When Paul and David came across the bandstand one day, in storage in the vacant lot, they thought it had been discarded and set about helping the village to dispose of the structure. Wielding a couple of small axes, they had succeeded in making firewood of most of the bandstand before someone came along and stopped them. My father and Uncle Henry paid for the damage, of course, and it was considered that the boys did not deserve punishment because they had meant well. The cost of the bandstand must have been more than justified in my father's opinion by his many laughs when he told and retold the story.

JUSTINE

Justine, the youngest child, was a pretty little girl with brown eyes and brown hair. All four of us girls had brown eyes and hair like our father, and both boys had blue-green eyes and blond hair. (Our mother had blue eyes and brown hair.) Because we girls looked so much like our father, a number of people in the community believed that we girls were his only children. I remember Justine as being rather quiet, although not as quiet as Ginger. She and Paul were close companions although she usually stayed out of trouble. Compared with Paul, the other five of us were relatively trouble-free.

THE PERFECT MAN

My mother adored my father. She called him "the doctor" and thought he was perfect in every way—well, except for one small fault. Here's what Arnold Gadow had to say about that: "He had one fault that I thought wasn't good. When I worked in the (Goblirsch General) store, he would always come in the back and buy snuff from me. It was 10 cents a can and came in a roll of eight. He called it 'dynamite'."

HUNTING

With a large family of children and his active medical practice to occupy him, he had little time for fishing, although I remember his taking all of us children fishing on several occasions. We caught bullheads, and he was kept busy baiting our lines and removing the fish we caught. He continued to hunt pheasants, sometimes out of season, which my mother, who was an expert wild game cook, would prepare. Paul recalled, "Going hunting (with Dad) was a big highlight for me. Never for ducks, but yes, for pheasants. Al and I were the road spotters. He would come home late in the afternoon and we would go out with him. We would spot the pheasants from the car and Dad would shoot them. I had a pretty good eye. He usually got his limit. It was illegal, of course, but they tasted good." In addition to it not being pheasant hunting season most of the time, it was probably also against the law to shoot from the car, but those pheasants were indeed tasty.

GARDENS

We didn't have a garden; we had gardens. One garden did not seem to offer enough scope to such an avid gardener as my father. My mother grew flowers. She had iris and peonies around the house, and in the plot below the backyard were hollyhocks, sweet peas, morning glories, sweet William, larkspur, and some rather spectacular oriental poppies that were the envy of her friends. He grew vegetables, sometimes trying out varieties that were unusual in Minnesota. We had lettuce, radishes, onions, green peas, beans, carrots, parsnips, cucumbers, cabbage, kale, kohlrabi, asparagus, rhubarb, ground cherries, and tomatoes. The tomato plants were fostered indoors and set out, when there was no longer danger of frost, in little box frames made from butter containers—the frames protected them from "cut worms." One year he planted peanuts and another year, snow peas. In addition to the garden near our house, he had another garden several blocks away for squash, sweet corn, potatoes, cantaloupe, watermelons, and strawberries. Alongside it was an orchard with plum and apple trees. We all helped in the garden, at least we thought we were helping, but we were probably more hin-

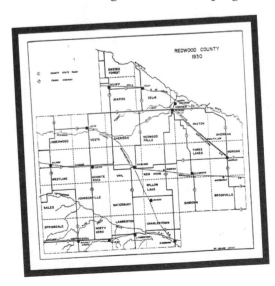

Fig. 43: *Map of Redwood County in 1930, showing Wabasso situated in Vail township in almost the exact center of the county, the railroad track and county roads intersecting the village.*

drance than help. We also helped prepare the fresh produce for the table and for canning. There was so much that we spent most of our summers, or so it seemed to me, canning. I'm sure my mother had in mind that we were kept under her eye and out of trouble.

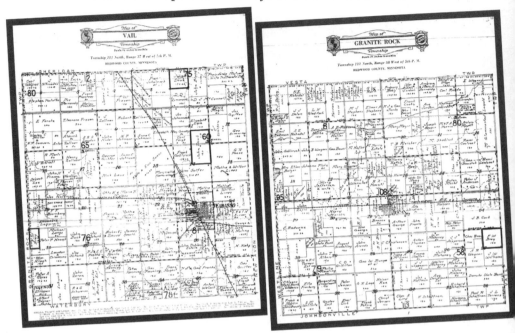

(From Left to Right)

Fig. 44: *Map of Vail township in 1930, showing the smaller portion of Dr. F. W. Brey's farm located at the extreme western edge of the township (section 30). The John E., Daub, homestead (sections 11 and 14) is situated about two miles north of the village beside the county road, and the John E. Daub III farm (section 2) about two miles farther north, along the north border of the township. The Frank Goblirsch farm (section 14) was originally homesteaded by Theodore Daub.*

Fig. 45: *Map of Granite Rock township, showing the larger portion of the F. W. Brey farm located along the eastern edge of the township (section 25).*

THE FARM

My father's fascination with growing things never flagged, and this was exemplified by his compelling and long-lasting interest in his farm. He had purchased the farm [Figures 43-45], located approximately four miles west of Wabasso, early in his career, before he was married. The mortgage was held by a widow who lived across the street from us in Wabasso, and the annual payments were made with whatever income the farm earned that year. We never lived on the farm, but my father often collected the lot of us children and took us along on his frequent visits. The farm was occupied by tenants who lived in the farmhouse and cultivated the land, the Klabunde family for many years and later the Siekora family. My father felt that the job not only offered work for the tenant farmer but also supplied a home for the tenant's family.

POLITICS

His favorite political party was the Farmer-Labor party, which later became the Democratic Farmer Labor (DFL) party. In 1938 he had the honor of introducing the gubernatorial candidate, Elmer Benson, on an outdoor platform in the center of the village [Figure 46]. After the candidate completed his address, a noon dinner was served by the "hotel girls" in the Commercial Hotel.

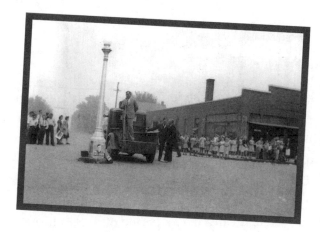

Fig. 46: *Photograph of Dr. Frank W. Brey introducing Minnesota gubernatorial candidate Elmer Benson at a political rally in Wabasso in 1938. This was probably the last photograph taken of him.*

THE DEPRESSION

The Great Depression, beginning with the stock market crash in 1929 and continuing throughout most of the 1930s, was a difficult time for many, but as a child I was quite unaware that times were hard. We always had enough to eat, and my parents never discussed the depression. I'm sure my father was never paid for much of the work he did. In later years my mother mentioned that he came home some evenings and told her that he had not been paid one cent that day. She also mentioned that she had not had a single new item of clothing for ten years. People who lived in villages and small towns probably felt the depression less than people who lived in urban areas because almost everyone had a garden and sometimes even a few chickens. Living was cheaper, and it was not as important to dress well.

Homeless men, referred to as "bums" or "hobos," passed through Wabasso as they did through other railroad towns. They hitched rides on the train boxcars and hung out in groups in "hobo jungles" near the railroad station, where they would build bonfires and boil coffee in tin cans over the fires. The men, who often knocked on doors, asking for handouts, were never sent away hungry from our home. They were not given money but were asked to perform a small service such as bringing in firewood in exchange for food. They were served at a picnic table in the backyard with whatever was on hand for our meal or, if nothing else was available, a plate of eggs, bacon, and fried potatoes, along with bread, butter, and coffee.

A FAMILY SECRET

That every family has at least one skeleton in its closet is common wisdom. I would have sworn that mine had none, since all the members of my family, in my opinion, were so honest and upright that they came close to being bland and uninteresting. Imagine our astonishment when my sister Ann and I recently came upon evidence preserved among my father's papers that many years ago a relative with whom he had had a business relationship had systematically, over a period of years, cheated him out of thousands of dollars. The document, the report of an audit carried out by a Minneapolis firm of accountants, concluded that a large amount of money had been embezzled from a business in which my father was the owner and a silent partner.

Discovery of this loss answered a question that had always puzzled me. Why were we so badly off financially after my father died? He had practiced medicine for 30 years, eleven of those years as an unmarried man, and even though his fees were low and frequently uncollected, he should have accumulated a fair amount of money. My mother was not at all extravagant. On the contrary, she was extremely frugal and spent very little money on herself and the household. I could not help thinking, fifty or so years later, that the money would have made a difference to the family, especially to my mother, who was left a widow with six children to educate. There was no social security in those days. For myself, I probably would not have had to hold an outside job through my years in medical school and would not have had to drop out after my second year to earn the tuition for my third and fourth years.

My mother must have known about the financial loss, of course, but neither she nor my father ever as much as hinted at the betrayal or indicated by any change of attitude whom the involved family member was. Our extended family gatherings continued, and we all spent holidays together as before. My parents had a firm policy of not revealing confidential matters, which was integral to their medical and nursing training. Although I often heard my parents discussing medical matters at the dinner table, for example, they never named names when talking about cases or patients. In this instance, they must have felt that there was nothing to gain by the disruption and acrimony that revealing the secret would have caused within the family.

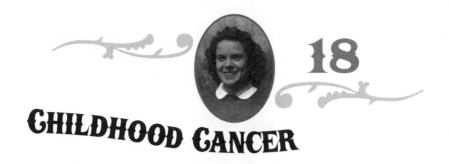

CHILDHOOD CANCER

18

When people learn that I am a pediatric hematologist/oncologist, they often say, "My, that must be depressing," or, "That must be so hard for you." Actually, there is good reason to feel optimistic about childhood cancer. Much of the pioneer work in treating cancer was done in children and the outlook for childhood cancer today is really quite positive. Childhood cancer is rare, with cancers in persons under 21 years of age making up only one or two percent of all cancers. An estimated 10,000 children under the age of 20 years are diagnosed with cancer in the U.S. each year. Cancer is the leading cause of death from disease after accidents in U.S. children age 1-14 years. Cancer is also the leading cause of death from disease after accidents, homicide, and suicide in U.S. adolescents age 15-19 years.

CHILDHOOD CANCER CURES

The current cure rate for childhood cancer is one of the notable medical successes of our time. At present the overall cure rate for childhood and adolescent cancer is 75-76 percent, and the rate is even higher for some specific types of childhood cancer. For example, the five-year survival for acute lymphoblastic leukemia, the most common childhood cancer, is 82 percent; for Wilms tumor of the kidney, 92 percent; and for thyroid carcinoma, 100 percent. One in 1,000 persons of all ages and one in 570 young adults between 20 and 34 years of age are childhood cancer survivors. At the present time there are approximately 300,000 survivors of childhood cancer in the U. S.[10]

When I joined the staff of the Oklahoma University Hospital and started working with child cancer patients in 1961, the outlook for them was indeed grim. The overall survival rate in the U.S. was 28%, and only a few forms of childhood cancer were curable by surgery or radiation. Acute lymphoblastic leukemia, the most common form of childhood cancer, was invariably fatal although we could achieve remissions, that is, periods when there was no evidence of disease. Children with solid tumors could sometimes be treated effectively with surgery and/or radiation, but it was necessary to tell the parents of every child with acute lymphoblastic leukemia that the child would die. Chemotherapy was just coming into use. The first effective cancer chemotherapy agent, aminopterin, had been introduced in 1948, and prednisone was recognized as an active drug against leukemia in 1949 and 1950. The only hope we could offer was that a true cure might be found in the interim if we could buy enough time with a series of remissions.

It gradually became clear that longer remissions were being obtained by starting treatment with large doses of multiple drugs and not waiting for relapses; and by the time I began seeing children with cancer in Michigan, cures were being claimed by St. Jude's Center for Childhood Cancer in Memphis, Tennessee. Even then, it was a long time before the concept of curing leukemia became generally accepted.

SOUTHWEST ONCOLOGY GROUP

Because Oklahoma was a member of the Southwest Oncology Group (SWOG), I was fortunate to get to know a number of pediatric hematologists/oncologists at other institutions in the area, and I learned a lot from my colleagues. They were, without exception, helpful in a kindly way, and I did not hesitate to telephone Margaret P. Sullivan, MD, or Wataru W. Sutow, MD, both at the M. D. Anderson Hospital in Houston, Texas, or Teresa J. Vietti, MD, at Washington University in St. Louis, Missouri, when I needed advice about patient care.

SWOG, POG, AND COG

Oklahoma was a member of the pediatric division of SWOG (Southwest Oncology Group), which later became POG (Pediatric Oncology Group). Many if not most of our meetings were held in New Orleans, and Fran came along on occasion, so that we were both able to enjoy visiting that beautiful city. The remarkable advances in the treatment of childhood cancer resulted from cooperative clinical trials, in which a group of institutions pooled their knowledge and treated large numbers of patients according to protocols, thus testing the effectiveness of individual drugs or of treatment regimens. POG and CCSG (Children's Cancer Study Group) later joined to become the present COG (Children's Oncology Group). COG protocols are used today to treat approximately 90% of all pediatric cancers in the U.S.

PATIENTS I REMEMBER

The very first child that I diagnosed with acute lymphoblastic leukemia was a pretty little five-year-old girl with beautiful blonde hair. One of the side effects of chemotherapy is hair loss, and she was distressed while under treatment to find herself totally bald. Her family was very poor. Because she was receiving welfare, as were most of the children in the Children's Hospital in Oklahoma City, I went to her welfare officer and asked for a wig. He had never had such a request before, and he refused, saying, "Why should we pay for a wig, when she's going to die anyway?" I continued to press for the wig, and eventually he produced a little blond wig made of some material that seemed to be very much like straw. It was stiff and irritating and scratched her tender scalp so badly that she could not wear it. Eventually her own hair grew back, temporarily, because she did not survive. At that time we had no social worker, who would be part of the treatment team in later years, to help us with such matters. Supplying a wig for hair loss is now a routine health care expense for any child patient with cancer.

A second memorable patient was an eight-year-old boy who had been diagnosed elsewhere with acute leukemia, followed by a complete remission, in which no evidence of leukemia could be found. It had been known for some time that such spontaneous remissions could occur, usually resulting from an "insult" of some sort, such as an infection, blood transfusion, surgical procedure, or for no apparent reason. Spontaneous remissions were of great interest to oncologists because it was thought that they could offer a clue to treatment and even cure. For this reason there was a great deal written about them in the medical literature in those early days when we had so little to offer cancer patients. This boy's remission occurred after chicken pox, but the infection left his face and entire body covered with ugly, discolored keloids. A keloid is a raised scar from an excess amount of tissue at the healing site that occurs when healing is abnormal. I saw him for the first time at the University of Oklahoma Medical Center after he relapsed. His parents had not been told that the remission would be only temporary, and they had believed him to be cured. Consequently, they were distraught when the leukemia recurred and he needed to be hospitalized again. He had a second short remission and again relapsed. Unfortunately, his parents abandoned him in the hospital about one week before he died, leaving this little boy to be comforted by strangers during the last hours of his life. I never knew why they chose such a cruel course of action; evidently they could not deal with their own emotions, perhaps because of his facial scarring and grotesque appearance. I was left with strong feelings of guilt because I felt that somehow I should have been able to convince them to help their son through his final days. Again, having a social worker as part of our team would have been immensely valuable.

My third interesting Oklahoma patient was one who seemed to have a near-miracle cure. In those days I always informed the parents of children with acute leukemia that there was no chance of cure, but I did not discourage them if they wanted to hope for a miracle. It was usual practice at that time to treat with an anti-leukemic drug and wait for a relapse before starting another anti-leukemic drug, attempting to achieve remission after remission, hoping to prolong the child's life as long as possible with the hope that a new curative treatment would come along in the meantime. A two-year-old boy with leukemia was enrolled on a protocol that called for three weeks of prednisone in full dosage and a fourth week in which the dose was gradually decreased. He went into a remission as expected, and the plan was to start another drug as soon as he relapsed. His leukemia never recurred. He had been enrolled on a SWOG protocol aimed at defining just how effective prednisone was. Such a protocol would have been impossible to use later, as more chemotherapeutic agents became available and treatment schedules for leukemia became more complex. His diagnosis was confirmed by my SWOG colleagues and his case was reported in the medical literature because a cure from such minimal treatment was unheard of.[11] Years later, after I had left Oklahoma, his case was again reported, this time as a 24-year-old man in good health.[12]

REFERENCES

10. Reaman, G. H. Pediatric Cancer II. In *2005 Annual Meeting Summaries,* Amer Soc Clin Oncol, 41st Annual Meeting, May 13-17, 2005, pp196-200.

11. Vietti, T. J., Sullivan, M. P., Berry, D. H., Haddy, T. B., Haggard, M. E., Blattner, R. J. The response of acute childhood leukemia to an initial and a second course of prednisone. *J Pediatr* 1965;66;18-26.

12. Fernbach, D. J. Natural history of acute leukemia. In *Clinical Pediatric Oncology,* 3rd edition, eds Sutow, W. W., Fernbach, D. J., Vietti, T. J., p 364.

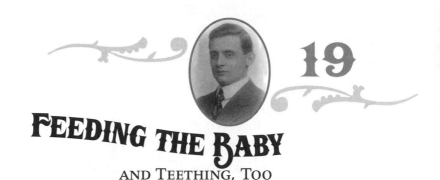

FEEDING THE BABY

AND TEETHING, TOO

Anticipatory guidance for raising infants and children was itself in its infancy in the early twentieth century. The University of Minnesota Medical School created a Department of Pediatrics in 1915, with Julius Parker Segwick as professor and chairman of the department. The diseases of children had previously been included under the Department of Internal Medicine. The American Academy of Pediatrics, which today sets standards for child feeding, rearing, and immunization practices, was not organized until the mid-1920s.

My father enjoyed caring for children, and many of his activities had to do with children. I am convinced that if he had specialized, which very few physicians did at that time, he would have been a pediatrician. An incident that happened during my childhood is an example of how he behaved toward children. One evening a small child, perhaps ten years old or so, whom I did not know, knocked on our front door. She was selling patent medicines. He invited her in and listened thoughtfully while she explained that the ointment (she called it a salve) would cure athlete's foot (fungus infection of the feet). I remember how scandalized I was—this little girl was telling my doctor father how to doctor!—but, of course, I said nothing. After she had finished her prepared speech, he bought a tin of ointment from her, thanked her for the purchase, and ushered her out the door. I never found out whether he knew the child or whether he used the ointment.

One of Arnold Gadow's anecdotes also helps illustrate how Dr. Brey felt about children. He wrote: "I remember your father from my growing up years. It was in 1918 during the war that we were ill with influenza. Most everyone had it at that time and many died. The school was shut down for some time. It was at that time that the Dr. came to our house and treated us. All the family had the influenza but my father. The Dr. walked to our home which he did so often for all the people in Wabasso. It was at that time I admired his watch and he took it off the chain and gave it to me. It was an open faced watch. It was a gold watch and my brother used it on the job when he worked on the railroad with my father."

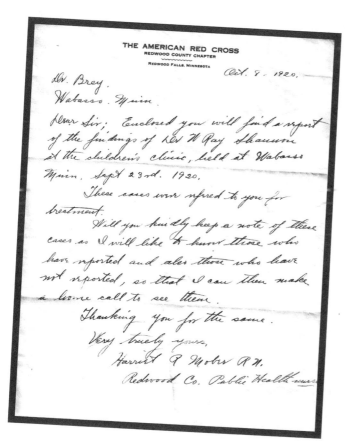

Fig. 47: *Letter from American Red Cross nurse Harriet R. Mober, R. N., to Dr. Brey, dated October 8, 1920.*

AN AMERICAN RED CROSS CHILDREN'S CLINIC

Found among his papers is a referral letter [Figure 47] hand-written by public health nurse Harriet R. Mober, R.N., from the Redwood County Chapter of the American Red Cross, in which she relayed to him the results of a children's clinic held in Wabasso on September 23, 1920, and asked him to follow up on the children who had been seen in the clinic. The compassionate concern of the public health nurse and physician, Dr. W. Ray Shannon, for their small patients is obvious. The nurse's meticulous report would serve as a model for any public health clinic today. She neatly listed Dr. Shannon's findings and recommendations on two extra pages, and referred the patients to "family physician—Dr. Brey." Ms. Mober wrote, "These cases are referred to you for treatment," and she further asked Dr. Brey to keep a record of the patients so that she could make "a home call to see" those who had not complied with the referral.

Twenty-one children, ranging in age from four months to five years of age, were seen in the clinic that day [Table 6]. Eighteen children were from Wabasso, one child was from Lamberton, and two had Redwood Falls addresses (they probably lived on farms). Nine children, who appeared to be well and evidently required no specific treatment, had tonic prescribed—Ph and CLO. Clearly, CLO is cod liver oil, but what is Ph? Does Ph refer to pasteurized honey, which, I have been told, was a popular pick-me-up or restorative at that time? A four month old baby girl had "food prescribed"—15 oz. milk, 15 oz. cereal water, $3\frac{1}{2}$ tablespoon sugar—6 oz. (to be given) every 4 hours, along with tonic Ph and CLO and a v. p. test. Another baby girl, also four months old, had "food prescribed—oatmeal mixture & milk 6 oz. (to be given)—five times a day or every four hours," along with tonic Ph and CLO. Tonsillectomies were recommended for four children, one with "ear trouble," and removal of both tonsils and adenoids was recommended for four more. A one-year-old boy had a "hernia straped [sic] by doctor," and a three year old girl had "surgical treatment" recommended for "congenital cleft palate."

TABLE 6. *Results of Children's Clinic, September 23, 1920, in Wabasso, Minnesota. Dr. W. Ray Shannon's findings and treatment recommended to family physician, Dr. Brey.*

Child	Age	Address	Treatment Recommended
P. T.	1 yr +	Redwood Falls	Tonic—Ph & CLO
R. A.	2 yrs +	Lamberton	" Ph & CLO
H. S.	1 yr +	Wabasso	" Ph & CLO
F. B.	7 mos -	"	" Ph & CLO
J. T.	1 yr +	"	" Ph & CLO
H. B.	1 yr +	"	" Ph & CLO
D. S.	1 yr +	"	" Ph & CLO
L. T.	2 yrs +	"	" Ph & CLO
R. P.	4 mos	"	" Ph & CLO and V. P. test
			Food prescribed, 15 oz milk 15 oz of cereal water 3½ tablespoon sugar 6 oz q 4 hr
E. T.	4 mos	Wabasso	Tonic—Ph & CLO
			Food prescribed, oatmeal mixture @ milk 6 oz 5 times a day or q 4 hr
C. S.	3 yrs +	Wabasso	Removal of Tonsils
L. B.	7 yrs +	"	" " "and Adenoids
A. S.	2 yrs +	"	" " "
C. Z.	3 yrs +	Redwood Falls	" " "and Adenoids
J. G.	5 yrs +	Wabasso	" " "
S. T.	2 yrs +	"	Ear trouble, Removal of Tonsils
G. T.	4 yrs +	"	"""" and Adenoids
L. T.	6 yrs +	"	" " " and Adenoids
L. C.	1 yr +	"	Hernia straped [sic] by Doctor
F. W.	2 yrs +	"	Tonic—Ph & CLO
I. M. H.	3 yrs -	"	Surg treatment (Congenital Cleft Palate)

FEEDING THE BABY

Dr. Brey must have been inspired by the demands of raising his own brood of children to write, most likely with assistance from my mother, the small booklet entitled *Feeding the Baby: The Right Food for the Baby and the Growing Child* [Figure 48a-f]. My sister Ann remembered that the feeding instructions were originally on a legal size sheet of paper,

Fig. 48a-f:
Feeding the Baby: The Right Food for the Baby and the Growing Child by Dr. Frank W. Brey.

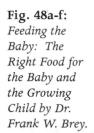
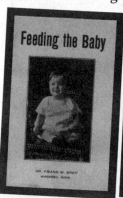
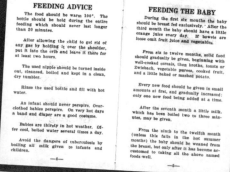
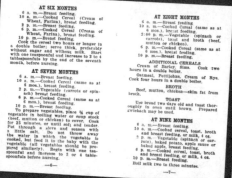
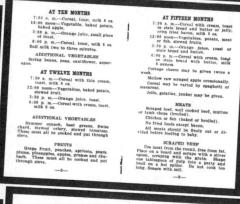
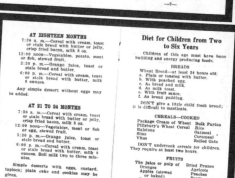

posted inside one of our kitchen cupboards and religiously followed. "The instructions were okayed at the Mayo Clinic," she told me, "and after being put into pamphlet form, a copy was given to every new mother." On the blue cover of the booklet is a photograph of my brother Al, looking the very model of an alert, healthy baby. Al, who appears to be about nine months old in the photograph, was born in 1925. The pamphlet is not dated, so it was probably printed in 1926 or 1927. The contents of his booklet are very similar to a set of undated instructions entitled *How to Feed the Baby* prepared for the Minnesota Public Health Association by the Northwestern Pediatric Society and endorsed by the Pediatric (Children's) Department of the Medical College of the University of Minnesota, which was found in somewhat bedraggled shape among his papers [Figure 49a,b]. Judging from its tattered appearance, it might have been the very sheet that Ann remembers seeing posted in our kitchen.

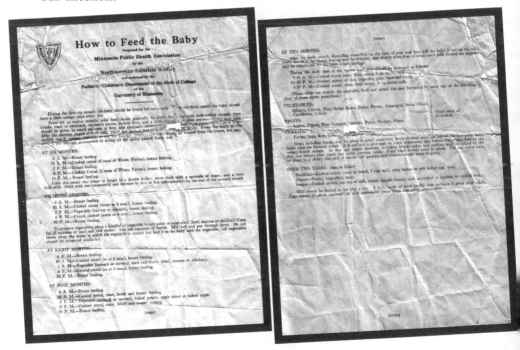

Fig. 49a,b: *How to Feed the Baby, prepared for the Minnesota Public Health Association by the Northwestern Pediatric Society and endorsed by the Pediatric (Children's) Department of the Medical College of the University of Minnesota.*

My father's feeding advice was not appreciably different from recommendations in vogue today although his reasons do not always coincide with modern thought. He did not mention vitamin supplementation, although orange juice was to be started as soon as breast feeding was discontinued. Nor did he mention infant immunization, which was not available at that time.

His instruction to breast feed for the first six months and delay feeding solid foods until then corresponds with current recommendations for normal infants. Admonitions to hold the bottle throughout the entire feeding and to offer boiled water several times each day during hot weather also correspond with current pediatric recommendations. He suggested that cow's milk should be gradually introduced after the seventh month, with a plan to discontinue breast feeding sometime between the ninth and twelfth months. He cautioned, however, that the milk must be boiled for two to three minutes to prevent tuberculosis. So important was this caution that it was mentioned in the section on general Feeding Advice and repeated three times, under the sections on Feeding the Baby, At Nine Months, and At Ten Months, presumably because parents might have become less vigilant as the child became more mature.

Under the section on Don'ts, the first listing in the pamphlet was, "Don't give coffee." There was good reason for this instruction because not all families gave their children milk. Among my schoolmates who lived on farms, it was not unknown for the parents to sell the milk from their cows and give their children coffee to drink.

Although a daily amount of orange juice was advised, its value as a source of vitamin C was not stated. Pasteurization of milk protected children from infection but presented a new danger, the possible development of scurvy. It had long been known that scurvy could be prevented by feeding as little as one ounce of orange juice daily. Therefore, orange juice was begun at ten months, as were fruits, after breast feeding was discontinued at nine months. "Strongly acid" fruits, not to be given to little children, are not defined; however, grapefruit was one of the recommended fruits. Mothers were encouraged not to throw away the water in which vegetables were cooked but to save it and feed it to the baby along with the vegetables. The reason for this, which is not mentioned, was so that the vitamins and minerals would be retained. Although cod liver oil was known to contain vitamins A and D, the pamphlet does not contain this information. I remember my father saying that forcing a child to take such terrible-tasting medicine amounted to cruelty to children. His own children were, however, given cod liver oil; it came in a brown bottle shaped like a fish. When halibut oil became available in gelatin capsules, my father switched enthusiastically to the capsules and we each took one every day during the winter. My cousin Belva Wilkinson recalled that a bowl of halibut capsules was placed on a side table near the front door as one entered our house.

Commercially prepared canned baby foods were not available. Mothers were advised to prepare strained foods by sieving, pureeing, and mashing cooked table fruits and vegetables for the baby. Apples and meat were scraped. Cooked cereals (cream of wheat, oatmeal, and farina), meat broths, jello, junket, tapioca, and plain blanc mange or cornstarch pudding could be served as is. The baby was to graduate to chopped, that is, finely cut or divided, foods at 15 months. In agreement with current American Academy of Pediatrics recommendations, new foods were to be given in small amounts at first and gradually increased, and only one new food was to be added at a time.

Fat was frowned upon, as it is today. Pastries (because of the fat), heavy salad dressings, and rich or fatty meats (such as pork) were proscribed. Fat was to be skimmed from broth. Fried foods were not allowed, except for bacon, which could be offered at 18 months if fried crisp so that all fat was removed.

Candy and intense sweets were not recommended. As children, we were not allowed to have candy, except for horehound and rock crystal candy, which were purchased at the drug store on rare occasions. We were not allowed to have pastries until we were five years old. Even then, the older children had to wait until the younger ones passed the five-year age mark, so that they would not be obliged to look on with envy while we ate foods that they were not allowed. (We older children resented this restriction.)

Salted, cured, or smoked meat or fish were listed under Don'ts, as they would be today because of the salt and nitrites they contain. Most modern pediatricians would probably disagree with the recommendation for cream on cooked cereal, butter on toast, and salt for seasoning the vegetables. Current thought would be to go lightly on all three.

TUBERCULOSIS

Tuberculosis, which continued to be a major cause of disability and death in the 1920s, was contracted from two main sources. The human strain, transmitted by respiratory droplets, lodged mainly in the lungs. The bovine strain, which is essentially not seen today, was transmitted through cow's milk and usually homed in on the bones or lymph nodes. Although not worthy of mention in the current American Academy of Pediatrics infectious disease handbook, because it has been essentially eliminated through effective public health measures, bovine tuberculosis was then a matter for serious concern. The spine was often affected, resulting in kyphosis, or "humpback." Pasteurization of milk, by heating milk to 145 degrees Fahrenheit for 15 minutes or to 170 degrees for a few minutes, was known to kill bacteria and thereby prevent tuberculosis. A method of testing cattle for tuberculosis, so that diseased cows could be culled from the herd, was available, but at that time there was no uniform or compulsory tuberculosis testing program. Rural families, who usually fed their children raw milk from their own cows (if they fed their children milk at all), sometimes resisted having the cows tested because a positive result meant that a portion of or the entire herd would have to be destroyed.

My father was so concerned about the transmission of bovine tuberculosis that he established his own small herd of two carefully tested cows from which we obtained our milk. The cows were stabled below our gardens, about a block south of our house, and were cared for by Henry (Hank) Gores. Hank, an elderly retired farmer, came faithfully every morning and evening to feed and milk the cows. For his work, he was paid ten dollars each week. At around that same time, the standard payment to our "hired girl" was fifty cents each week in addition to her room and board. Girls from farms were often hired by families living in town under such an arrangement so that the girls could attend the Wabasso High School.

THE DEVELOPMENT OF BABY'S TEETH

He also published a small booklet on teething entitled *The Development of Baby's Teeth* [Figure 50a-d]. Although undated, the booklet must have been written about the same time as the feeding pamphlet. It states that "The baby's teething causes the mother much anxiety and worry, which could be largely avoided if mothers were better informed." Care of the teeth by brushing (each evening) and regular visits to the dentist (yearly) are advocated, and a strong case is made that "care of the teeth in childhood is many times repaid in later life."

We were fortunate enough to be the recipients of excellent dental care in childhood. Our parents' dental care had been carried out by Dr. C. L. Lynn, until he left Wabasso in 1925. Dr. H. A. Young was the dentist in Wabasso for the next few years, followed by Dr. A. J. McLean, who was our family dentist from 1928 through the 1930s.

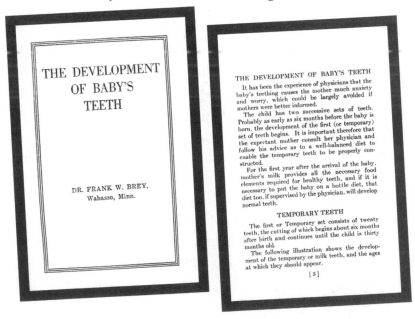

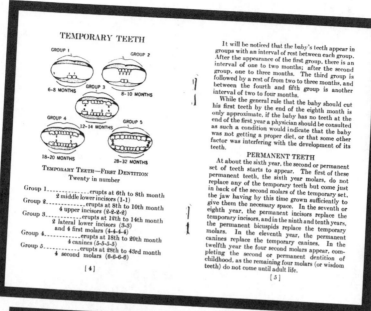

TEMPORARY TEETH

TEMPORARY TEETH—FIRST DENTITION
Twenty in number

Group 1............erupts at 6th to 8th month
2 middle lower incisors (1-1)
Group 2............erupts at 8th to 10th month
4 upper incisors (2-2-2-2)
Group 3............erupts at 12th to 14th month
2 lateral lower incisors (3-3)
and 4 first molars (4-4-4-4)
Group 4............erupts at 18th to 20th month
4 canines (5-5-5-5)
Group 5............erupts at 28th to 43rd month
4 second molars (6-6-6-6)

[4]

It will be noticed that the baby's teeth appear in groups with an interval of rest between each group. After the appearance of the first group, there is an interval of one to two months; after the second group, one to three months. The third group is followed by a rest of from two to three months, and between the fourth and fifth group is another interval of two to four months.

While the general rule that the baby should cut his first teeth by the end of the eighth month is only approximate, if the baby has no teeth at the end of the first year a physician should be consulted as such a condition would indicate that the baby was not getting a proper diet, or that some other factor was interfering with the development of its teeth.

PERMANENT TEETH

At about the sixth year, the second or permanent set of teeth starts to appear. The first of these permanent teeth, the sixth year molars, do not replace any of the temporary teeth but come just in back of the second molars of the temporary set, the jaw having by this time grown sufficiently to give them the necessary space. In the seventh or eighth year, the permanent incisors replace the temporary incisors, and in the ninth and tenth years, the permanent bicuspids replace the temporary molars. In the eleventh year, the permanent canines replace the temporary canines. In the twelfth year the four second molars appear, completing the second or permanent dentition of childhood, as the remaining four molars (or wisdom teeth) do not come until adult life.

[5]

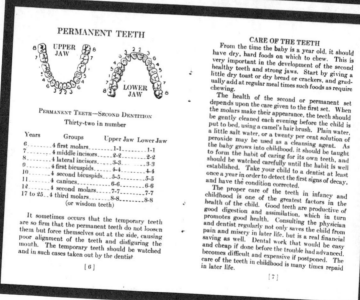

PERMANENT TEETH

PERMANENT TEETH—SECOND DENTITION
Thirty-two in number

Years	Groups	Upper Jaw	Lower Jaw
6	4 first molars	1-1	1-1
7	4 middle incisors	2-2	2-2
8	4 lateral incisors	3-3	3-3
9	4 first bicuspids	4-4	4-4
10	4 second bicuspids	5-5	5-5
11	4 canines	6-6	6-6
12	4 second molars	7-7	7-7
17 to 25	4 third molars	8-8	8-8
	(or wisdom teeth)		

It sometimes occurs that the temporary teeth are so firm that the permanent teeth do not loosen them but force themselves out at the side, causing poor alignment of the teeth and disfiguring the mouth. The temporary teeth should be watched and in such cases taken out by the dentist

[6]

CARE OF THE TEETH

From the time the baby is a year old, it should have dry, hard foods on which to chew. This is very important in the development of the second healthy teeth and strong jaws. Start by giving a little dry toast or dry bread or crackers, and gradually add at regular meal times such foods as require chewing.

The health of the second or permanent set depends upon the care given to the first set. When the molars make their appearance, the teeth should be gently cleaned each evening before the child is put to bed, using a camel's hair brush. Plain water, a little salt water, or a twenty per cent solution of peroxide may be used as a cleansing agent. As the baby grows into childhood, it should be taught to form the habit of caring for its own teeth, and should be watched carefully until the habit is well established. Take your child to a dentist at least once a year in order to detect the first signs of decay, and have the condition corrected.

The proper care of the teeth in infancy and childhood is one of the greatest factors in the health of the child. Good teeth are productive of good digestion and assimilation, which in turn promotes good health. Consulting the physician and dentist regularly not only saves the child from pain and misery in later life, but is a real financial saving as well. Dental work that would be easy and cheap if done before the trouble had advanced, becomes difficult and expensive if postponed. The care of the teeth in childhood is many times repaid in later life.

[7]

Fig. 50a-d: *The Development of Baby's Teeth by Dr. Frank W. Brey.*
(Fig. 50a,b on previous page)

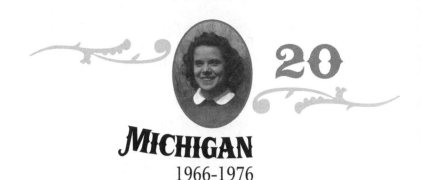

MICHIGAN
1966-1976

We left Oklahoma in 1966 with great reluctance, and Fran became chairman of the Department of Physiology at Michigan State University. MSU, which was already a large university, was adding a new medical school and it was his job to coordinate the teaching of physiology not only to the medical students but also to the students in other colleges, including veterinary medicine, agriculture, liberal arts, and others. A positive feature of the move was finding relatives in East Lansing, my mother's sister, Aunt Helen Taylor, her husband, Uncle Tom Taylor, and their youngest child, Jim, who was about the age of our children. They became good friends and had fun together. It was a difficult move, especially for Rick, who was in high school, and Carol, who was in the eighth grade. We felt that the public schools in Michigan were better, but the schools and therefore the classes were much bigger and more impersonal.

Our wonderful housekeeper, Mrs. Leslie, had been having some trouble with chest pains when she decided not to come with us but to retire. Nana was by then living with a daughter in Canada, and she visited us once in Michigan. Although she never once mentioned it to us, we heard later that her chest pains had been increasing in intensity. Sadly, she died soon after that visit. This was before the advent of anti-lipid medications, bypass surgery, and medicated stents for coronary occlusive disease. We hired Mrs. Holey to keep house and supervise Alice and the two older children after school.

We lived in East Lansing, a suburb of Lansing and the home of Michigan State University. I joined the Division of Child Health in the Michigan Department of Public Health, which is located in Lansing, the state capital. My chairman, Dr. Gerald Rice, was a good supervisor and it was a congenial department to work in.

MICHIGAN STATE UNIVERSITY

Because my public health job for the state was purely administrative, however, I welcomed an opportunity to join the Department of Human Development and Pediatrics in the MSU medical school because it would allow me to start seeing patients again. The pediatric department, called the Department of Human Development, was chaired by Dr. William Weil. Bill had been a student at the University of Minnesota, a year or so behind me, and had also been an intern at the Minneapolis General Hospital when I was there. Bill's wife, V (Velma), was at the MGH, too. She came there as a newly-hired nurse-anesthetist, and the news went quickly around the hospital grapevine, "The new nurse-anesthetist in the operating room is beautiful!" We all took what opportunity we could to go past the doors and have a look. The next bit of news was, "Bill Weil is going to ask her for a date!" Later we heard, "She said yes!" After that I heard no more about the romance until Fran and I moved to East Lansing and met Bill's wife, V.

PEDIATRIC HEMATOLOGY/ONCOLOGY

Again, I was the only pediatric hematologist/oncologist, and this time I was starting a new subspecialty division with a need for special laboratory tests in a department that was itself new. I was fortunate to again have close collaborators in the internal medicine department. Drs. Anthony J. Bowdler, Earl Campbell, and L. George Surhland were especially helpful. We used the three community hospitals in Lansing as well as MSU's student health service in East Lansing; this required "learning the ropes" in each hospital. Traveling from one hospital to another in Lansing took up a good deal of the faculty members' time. In addition, we were required to drive to towns around the state, for example, Grand Rapids, to teach MSU students who were deployed there. I began as an assistant professor and was later promoted to associate professor. During my time at MSU there were never enough patients to allow me to join one of the pediatric cancer clinical trials groups, but after I left, the number of patients increased and the department was able to join the Children's Cancer Chemotherapy Group (CCSG).

CHILDHOOD CANCER

More chemotherapeutic agents became available, and the treatment of childhood cancer continued to improve. Treating acute lymphoblastic leukemia involved a complicated protocol, administering a number of drugs simultaneously and in sequence by mouth and by the intravenous route, as well as preventive radiation and/or intrathecal chemotherapy to prevent leukemic infiltration of the brain and spinal cord. Intrathecal drugs are administered by placing a needle into the lower spinal canal and injecting the dose directly into the spinal fluid. In recent years cranial radiation is used for treatment only if the brain and spinal cord are involved and is not considered necessary or desirable for prevention because damage to the brain can occur. While I was at MSU, pediatric oncologists began for the first time to talk about "curing" acute lymphoblastic leukemia. I was pleased to be able to tentatively offer this possibility to parents of several children who remained in complete remission for two years or longer, and even more pleased to observe that their outcomes were good.

Although I became very busy, a second pediatric hematologist/ oncologist was never hired while I was at MSU. The local pediatricians were very supportive, however, and they were extremely helpful to me. All of my patients were seen in consultation with their private physicians, who continued to share in their care, sometimes arranging hospitalization or consultation with other specialists if needed, diagnosing and treating common infections, and sometimes administering intravenous and even intrathecal cancer chemotherapy.

SABBATICAL LEAVE

In 1972 Fran and I went to Aachen, Germany on his sabbatical leave from MSU. The sabbatical leave is standard at major universities, sabbatical referring to every seven years. Teachers in schools of higher education are granted this year, usually at half salary, so that they can go elsewhere for a year of study and bring back new ideas to their school. Since I had been at MSU for fewer than seven years, I was not eligible for a sabbatical leave, and instead, my department granted me a one year's leave without salary. Alice went with us; she was 14 years old when we left and 15 when we returned. Rick and Carol stayed behind because they were both in college, but they came to visit us at Christmas time. Fran studied at the Techniche Hohschule, and his sponsor, Dr. Gerlach, arranged for me to work at the Stadt Krankenhaus, the city hospital. Alice attended the Victoria Schule, a high school for college-bound girls. She could have gone to a nearby school for children of U.S. military personnel, but she preferred to attend the German school. She did very well and became a special friend of some charming German girls. She missed her first year of high school in East Lansing, and Fran and I were very pleased when the East Lansing High School accepted the credits earned in Aachen after her return. In Germany we were treated most graciously by everyone we dealt with and our experience there was most pleasant. This was especially gratifying because although World War II had ended with Germany's defeat only a quarter of a century earlier, there seemed to be no hard feelings on the part of anyone we came in contact with.

CHILDREN'S EDUCATION

Our children grew up. Rick completed his undergraduate work at St. Olaf College in Northfield, Minnesota, and went on to medical school at MSU. Carol, after spending two years at Northwestern University, transferred to MSU and got her degree in fine arts. Alice decided to leave high school after her junior year and was admitted early to the University of Michigan. Starting in the middle of her sophomore year, she worked her way through college and graduate school and obtained a Ph.D. in physical chemistry with a second major in anthropology.

LEAVING MICHIGAN

When Fran received an offer to chair the department of physiology in a new medical school, the Uniformed Services University of the Health Sciences in Bethesda, Maryland, which was sponsored by the Department of Defense, he was intrigued by the idea of again helping to start a new medical school. Our children were either in college or had completed their higher education, so when he accepted the offer, they did not move to the Washington, D.C., area with us.

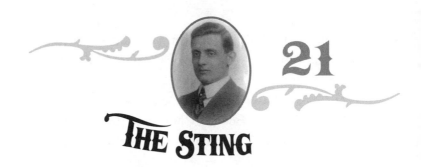

THE STING

arcotics and intoxicants were for all practical purposes unregulated until the Harrison Anti-narcotic Act, passed in 1914, became effective on March 1, 1915.[13,14] In 1920, the Eighteenth Amendment to the Constitution of the United States was ratified, and the Volstead Act, prohibiting "intoxicating liquors" that contained more than 0.5 percent alcohol, took effect. In 1933, the Twenty-first Amendment repealed prohibition. A 1,000 bed facility for men only, authorized by the United States Public Health Service through the Division of Mental Hygiene in the Office of the Surgeon General and known as the United States Narcotics Farm, was opened near Lexington, Kentucky, in 1935. Its purpose was "the segregation and confinement" of intractable drug addicts.

Although "heroic practice," with its vigorous use of blood letting, emetics, and cathartics, was declining at the end of the nineteenth and early in the twentieth century, there was still very little to offer in the way of specific remedies for diseases. Physicians aimed at relieving symptoms, that is, at making the patient feel better, rather than at curing the disease. In fact, so few diagnostic methods were available that it was not always possible to make a diagnosis. Among the drugs commonly used were opiates, cocaine, and alcohol. These drugs were frequently prescribed but were also easily obtainable over the counter without prescription.

Opium in the form of raw opium, laudanum, paregoric, heroin, and morphine effectively relieved pain and were useful for the suppression of cough and control of diarrhea. Opiates were prescribed for acute and chronic pain as well as insomnia and were so popular that by the 1890s a half million pounds of opium were being imported into the United States each year. Cocaine was not considered to be addictive, and this opinion continued to be prevalent among physicians well past the mid-twentieth century mark. Alcohol was frequently prescribed, usually as a tonic or stimulant, and was even given to infants and children.

Most medical historians believe that the majority of nineteenth century narcotics addicts belonged to the middle and upper classes and became addicted after being medicated by physicians. Health care professionals themselves, because of easy access to drugs, accounted for a substantial number of addicts. By the early twentieth century the idea that large numbers of addicts were of the middle and upper classes had changed, however, and the underworld was now thought to account for most cases of addiction. No occupation, nationality, race, or social class was exempt, but drug usage by then had come to be thought as more of a police problem than a medical issue.

ANNUAL INVENTORY

The Harrison Narcotic Law was intended to control the traffic in habit-forming drugs, especially opium and cocaine, by requiring all manufacturers, dealers, pharmacists, physicians, dentists, and veterinarians to be registered. Prescribing physicians registered with the district collector of internal revenue and renewed their licenses yearly for a fee of one dollar. Prescriptions included the patient's name and address, the physician's registry number, and the physician's signature. Copies or records of the prescription, which could not be refilled, were retained by the druggist. Drugs administered or dispensed by a physician while personally attending a patient did not need to be recorded, nor did preparations containing up to "2 grains of opium, $\frac{1}{4}$ grain of morphin [sic], 1/8 grain of heroin, or 1 grain of codein [sic]."

TABLE 7. *Partial list of Dr. Frank W. Brey's annual INVENTORY OF OPIUM, ETC reports for the decade from June 28, 1929, to June 21, 1938.*

Substance	1929	1932	1933	1934*	1935	1936	1938
Morphin [sic] Sulphate H. T. ¼ gr	48	140	24	6	450	350	450
Morphin [sic] Sulphate T. T. ¼ gr	30	-	-	-	-	-	-
Cocaine Hydrochloride H. T. ¼ gr	64	64	56	36	490	300	40
Cocaine Hydrochloride 1 gr dispensing tablets	-	31	11	5	-	-	-
Cocaine Hydrochloride 1 1/8 gr tablets	-	-	-	-	19	-	-
Cocaine Hydrochloride Powder 1/8 oz	1/8	1/8	-	-	-	-	-
Cocaine Hydrochloride Flakes	-	-	10 gr	-	1/8 oz	1/8 oz	-
Codeinae [sic] Sulphate H. T. ¼ gr	-	-	-	-	-	425	75
Codeinae [sic] Sulphate T. T. ¼ gr	200	-	-	-	-	-	-
Apomorphine Hydrochloride H. T. 1/10 gr	-	40	-	-	-	-	-

gr = grain(s); oz = ounce(s); H. T. = hypodermic tablet(s); T. T.= triturated tablet(s).
Trituration is reducing a solid to powder by rubbing, or making something homogeneous by mixing. A triturated drug is one rubbed with milk sugar (lactose).

* The inventory report for 1934 contains the handwritten notation, "Sent $1 cash."

My father (U.S. Registry Number 4530) duly cooperated with the Internal Revenue Service of the Treasury Department by submitting a yearly inventory of class 4 drugs in his possession [Table 7]. He described himself on the various forms as a "private practitioner" or "individual practitioner" and stated that his official position was "Practice of Medicine and Surgery." On one of his INVENTORY OF OPIUM, ETC submissions he noted, "Sent $1 cash." It is noteworthy that in 1935 he increased the quantity of narcotics on hand, but after that time kept no drugs for oral administration, only drugs that were used for hypodermic injection (beneath the skin) or for topical administration (applied to the skin or mucous membranes for local anesthesia, especially cocaine powder and flakes). These preparations were administered prior to and following surgical procedures, including tonsillectomy and adenoidectomy, incision and drainage of abscesses, and reduction and immobilization of fractures. I remember that he sometimes left several tablets of morphine, in a small, thin, glass tube, with terminally ill patients; the tablets were to be dissolved in a syringe and injected by a nurse or another qualified caretaker.

"OLD HABITUÉS"

In March, 1915, as the Harrison law was put into effect, the editors of the *Journal of the American Medical Association* explained to the practicing physicians of the United States that for "old habitués, persons suffering from painful and incurable diseases, and others to whom opium in some form is absolutely necessary—every physician knows of such cases—the physician...can prescribe whatever he sees fit."

In June, 1915, the editors responded to plaintive letters from physicians caring for addicted patients with further clarification of this law.[15] A. J. M., the only medical practitioner in his village, with the nearest drug store nine miles away, asked for guidance. Could he lawfully continue to supply an old (77 years of age) drug-dependent soldier with one grain of morphine daily? In answer, he was assured that "the Harrison law does not restrict the right of a physician to prescribe as he may see fit. It requires him to keep a record of any drug which he dispenses and requires the druggist to keep a record of prescriptions for such drugs." T. E. A., a physician practicing in Texas, likewise inquired about a patient who had been a habitué for years. "Shall I violate the law if I prescribe an opiate for him?" The answer: no.

It was not long before the official attitude changed. First, in March, 1919, the United States Supreme Court ruled against two defendants—

the physician for prescribing, the druggist for dispensing, narcotics— who were found guilty of maintaining an addict on narcotic drugs without intent to cure. Then, the American Medical Association, reflecting a widespread opinion on the part of the medical profession, came out against the so-called ambulatory treatment of narcotic addiction. This was a method, generally conceded to be ineffective, in which the patient was given a supply of the drug to take on his or her own, with a plan to reduce the dosage in decrements.

HIS OWN OLD HABITUÉ

Dr. Brey had his own old habitué to contend with, Mr. S. He faced the same difficult problem that other practitioners of the time faced: how should the chronically addicted patient of long standing be managed? Narcotic drugs, which induced blessed relief of pain, were at the same time dangerously addictive. He retained among his papers records that tell the sad story of his struggle to help this patient. The first indication of a dilemma was contained in a letter from Mayo Clinic consultant Dr. Lee W. Pollack dated October 10, 1928 [Figure 51]. In his letter, Dr. Pollack states that he saw Mr. S for the second

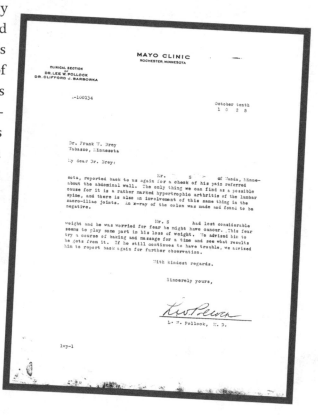

Fig. 51: *Letter from L. W. Pollock, M. D., at the Mayo Clinic, to Dr. Frank W. Brey dated October 10, 1928.*

time and was again unable to find a convincing physical cause for the patient's complaint of abdominal pain. (Dr. Pollack's initial referral letter is not available.)

The next letter in the series, dated May 5, 1932, is a copy of a letter [Figure 52] to Mr. O. A. H. de la Gardie, District Supervisor, Bureau of Narcotics, Minneapolis, from L. M. Wilcuts, Collector of Internal Revenue. Mr. Willcuts states that Dr. Brey's letter regarding a patient, Mr. S, and the patient's use of morphine is being referred to the Burieau of Narcotics for a reply. (A copy of Dr. Brey's letter is not included.)

The third letter retained among Dr. Brey's records, dated May 7, 1932, is a reply from J. P. Wall, Acting District Supervisor, United States Narcotic Service, Minneapolis, to Dr. Frank W. Brey "In re: Treatment of Addicts" [Figure 53]. The letter contains a stern admonition: "It

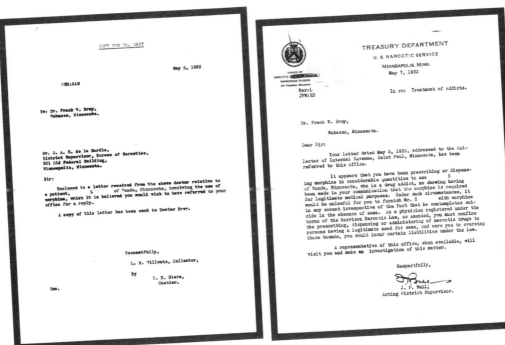

(From Left to Right)

Fig. 52: *Letter from L. M. Willcuts, Collector (of Internal Revenue?), to O. A. H. de la Gardie, Bureau of Narcotics, dated May 5, 1932.*

Fig. 53: *Letter from J. P. Wall, U. S. Narcotic Service, to Dr. Frank W. Brey, dated May 7, 1932.*

appears that you have been distributing or dispensing morphine in considerable quantities to one...drug addict, [with] no showing that the morphine is required for legitimate medical purposes. Under such circumstances it would be unlawful...irrespective of the fact that he contemplates suicide in the absence of same." No suggestion is offered for alternative management or disposition. Drug counseling was apparently not a viable option, and the United States Narcotic Farm near Lexington was not yet in existence. This rural physician and his patient were left on their own to try to cope with a serious problem.

Dr. Brey's final record regarding Mr. S is not a letter, but a death certificate, which confirms the 64-year-old patient's death on February 27, 1933, from self-inflicted 38 caliber gunshot wounds of the abdomen and head.

THE PHYSICIAN IN DANGER

Because physicians were known to maintain office supplies of narcotics and usually carried narcotics in their medical bags, they were at risk for the ever-present danger of physical assault by persons intent on stealing narcotics. They learned to be on guard, especially when making house calls, against being victimized. I remember that when I started practice in Arlington Heights, Dr. Leckband, a gracious older gentleman who was one of the medical practitioners in town, had a serious conversation with me about my personal safety. He advised me to look out, when I made housecalls at night, for people who wanted drugs. He described an instance when he had responded to a false call, and his automobile had been forced off the road by a couple of young men in another car. He had fortunately been able to get away. "Never go out on a call unless you know the family," he told me, "and, when in doubt, it wouldn't be amiss to alert the local police."

My mother told my sister Ann of a series of episodes; my father never discussed anything in our presence that might have alarmed us children. Fortunately, none of the episodes had serious consequences. He garaged his automobile at night in Jensen's garage, a local Ford garage that offered commercial parking. Ever wary at night, he customarily held the garage key in his right hand and a wrench in his left hand when he came for his car after hours. On one occasion, upon hearing an intruder, he quickly entered his car and drove off without stopping to investigate further or even to close the garage door. On another occasion, when driving down a country road on the way to a house call in the middle of the night, he encountered an automobile, facing toward him with its lights on, straddling the center of the two-lane road. He immediately pulled off the road into the ditch on the right, passed the stopped car, drove his car out of the ditch, and sped on his way. As with the previous episode, there was no firm indication of harmful intent, but caution told him not to wait around and find out.

Still another time, late one night, my mother called to him from their front bedroom window as he returned from a house call, to let him know that he should not come into the house but go directly to an emergency across the street. She relayed a telephone message from the family who lived there, asking him to proceed directly to their home because the grandmother, who lived with the family, was having an acute asthma attack. This request was not at all unusual, since she was a chronic asthmatic and he was often called there for that same reason. In fact, he was accustomed to making his way into the house without knocking, and going immediately to the elderly woman's bedroom to care for her. This time, however, he hesitated because the house was dark. As he approached their front porch, my mother, still looking out of the window, saw by the nearby streetlight that a person was standing behind a tree on the neighbor's front lawn. She called to my father again, and, fearful, he immediately headed home. Once inside his own house, he soon established that the telephone call had been faked.

Was it a "Sting" Operation?

In the fall of 1936, an unpleasant and ominous encounter in my father's Wabasso office initiated a chain of puzzling correspondence that ultimately reached the highest levels in Washington, D. C. [Figures

54-59]. This was an incident in which he must have been taken by surprise, and one that might have had serious consequences. The first letter [Figure 54], dated January 29, 1937, contains a request from George F. Sullivan, the United States Attorney, Department of Justice, St. Paul, for a "voluntary offer in compromise" of one hundred dollars, to be made by Dr. Brey because of "a rather serious violation of the Harrison Act." This was followed by a similar letter [Figure 55] dated February 16, 1937, from Joseph Bell, District Supervisor of the Bureau of Narcotics, Minneapolis, in which Dr. Brey was asked to fill out a report form.

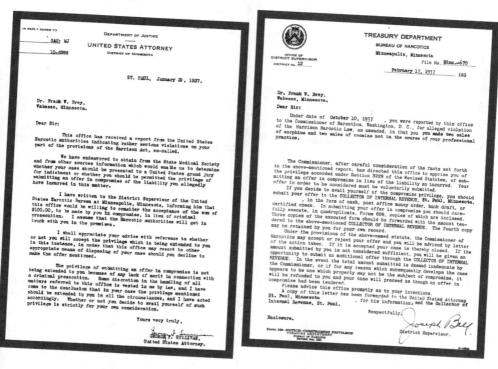

(From Left to Right)
Fig. 54: *Letter from George F. Sullivan, United States Attorney, to Dr. Frank W. Brey, dated January 29, 1937.*

Fig. 55: *Letter from Joseph Bell, Bureau of Narcotics, to Dr. Frank W. Brey, dated February 17, 1937.*

The report, dated February 18, 1937, from Dr. Brey to the Commissioner of Internal Revenue through the Collector of Internal Revenue,

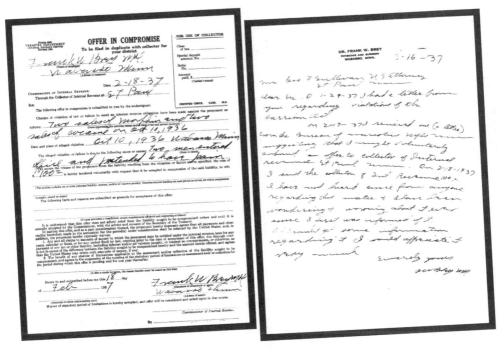

(From Left to Right)

Fig. 56: *Report form from Frank W. Brey, M. D., to Commissioner of Internal Revenue, dated February 18, 1937.*

Fig. 57: *Letter from Frank W. Brey, M. D., to George F. Sullivan, U. S. Attorney, dated March 16, 1937.*

St. Paul [Figure 56], asserts that on October 10, 1936, "two sales of morphin [sic] and two sales of cocaine" were made after "two men entered office and pretended to have pain." The abrupt, terse language of Dr. Brey's report gives it an angry tone. It is obvious that the men's claim was bogus; he clearly did not believe for a moment that they were both having pain. My father was a big, strong man, and he was nobody's patsy. Guns or other weapons are not mentioned, but the demands by the two strangers, most likely when he was alone in his office at night, must have been extremely intimidating. He would have been greatly concerned about the possibility of injury, not only to himself, but also to his wife and children at home.

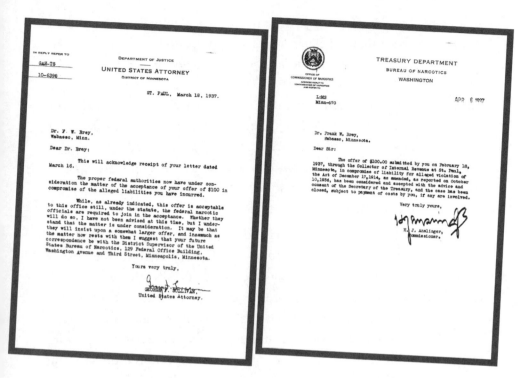

(From Left to Right)
Fig. 58: *Letter from George F. Sullivan, United States Attorney, to Dr. F. W. Brey, dated March 18, 1937.*

Fig. 59: *Letter from H. J. Anslinger, Commissioner, Bureau of Narcotics, to Dr. Frank W. Brey, dated April 6, 1937.*

One hundred dollars were paid by Dr. Brey on February 18, 1937. The payment was followed approximately one month later by a rather anxious inquiry [Figure 57] from Dr. Brey about his situation. A letter from Mr. Sullivan [Figure 58] on March 18, 1937 states that "this offer is acceptable to the state office" but would need final approval from the federal level. Correspondence concerning the incident was closed when the $100 was accepted in a letter [Figure 59] written April 6, 1937, from H. J. Anslinger, Commissioner of the Bureau of Narcotics, Washington, D.C.

Who were these mysterious men? What was the meaning of this enigmatic episode? My father would never voluntarily have sold drugs to anyone, but, clearly, he was at fault for failing to make an immediate report. To whom should he have reported? Wabasso had a constable and a justice of the peace. A word to either of them would have led to gossip and rumors. A telephone report to anyone would have had the same result, since the telephone operator routinely listened in on calls and was an inveterate gossip. Perhaps the best way to handle the situation would have been to send a letter to the U.S. Internal Revenue, to the same office that received his annual inventory. He probably waited, indecisive, and when there was no further word, decided not to pursue the matter, hoping that it would all go away.

In considering possible reasons for what transpired, the first and most obvious reason suggested to me is that someone in the Justice Department or Treasury Department created the situation in order to extort money. This possibility can be quickly dismissed because the affair involved too many people on too many levels, not only the state U.S. Attorney and the Bureau of Narcotics, but also the federal Treasury Department. Further, the amount of money, one hundred dollars, was too small to make such a complicated project worthwhile.

A second scenario was suggested to me by an employee of the Treasury Department in Washington, D.C., when I talked with him by telephone about what might have happened on October 10, 1936. That individual suggested that the two men who "entered office" might have been criminals who were arrested at a later date while carrying narcotics, the implication being that they could have tried to plea bargain by turning in the name of a country doctor they had preyed upon. This explanation seems unlikely, simply because most criminals would not have been satisfied with "two sales of morphin and two sales of cocaine." Surely they would have carried off the entire available supply of narcotics.

The third, most likely, possibility is that the two men were a team of government narcotics agents who were carrying out an undercover "sting" operation. If this is the correct reason, then the obvious question is, how did they choose their target? The Treasury Department employee with whom I spoke thought it likely that Dr. Brey's annual narcotics report could have been flagged because his inventory [Table

7] had increased by approximately tenfold in the preceding year. Against this reasoning is the fact that he did not subsequently decrease the amount kept on hand but continued to carry a large inventory of morphine. The Treasury Department employee suggested other reasons. An undercover operation could have been planned at random, he said, or it could have been instigated by a complaint, or by "suspicious activity in the area."

The possibility of "suspicious activity in the area" and the observation that Dr. Brey had increased his narcotics inventory in 1935 seem to lead to the only other place in the village where drugs would be available. My sister Ann remembered that he had decided to no longer send narcotics prescriptions to the local drug store because of what he called "irregularities" in the way prescriptions were being filled. The drug store proprietor, Bertha Schottenbauer, and my father had mutual respect for each other; I remember her as a tough but honest and upright woman, surely above suspicion. Because she was not trained as a pharmacist and could not dispense drugs, Bertha had hired a pharmacist named Hjalmer Larsen. According to Arnold Bauer's book, Mr. Larsen began working in Wabasso in 1928 and was still there in 1934, when the Bauer book about Wabasso was published. According to the Minnesota State Pharmacy Board Registration, on the other hand, Hjalmer Larsen listed Franklin, Minnesota, as his place of business from 1927 to 1934, and did not change it to Wabasso until 1935.

Examination of justice court, civil court, and indictment books of Redwood and Lyon Counties reveals that Hjalmer Larsen was convicted on November 22, 1913, in Lyon County Justice Court of operating an unlicensed drinking place. (Was he selling the pharmacy's ethyl alcohol on the side?) For this crime he was sentenced by Justice of the Peace K. Knudson to pay a $50 fine. Mr. Larsen's obituary, published in the *Cottonwood Current* newspaper on June 30, 1944, stated that he had served as pharmacist in nine towns, as follows: Granite Falls, Boyd, Benson, Milan, Graceville, Wabasso, Franklin, Bagley, and Clearbrook. The Minnesota State Pharmacy Board registration listed him as having had three additional places of business: Minneapolis, Cottonwood, and Morristown. The numbers add up to a total of 12 different towns. Interestingly, his obituary described him as a resident of Cottonwood who "had traveled extensively and had made the acquaintance of men in high places." It further stated, "His home contains priceless paintings, tapestries, pottery and other articles from the orient and elsewhere which the family prize most highly."

The full story of this enigma may never be known, but several pieces of the puzzle indicate entrapment of an honest, hard-working country doctor as the most likely explanation of this affair. It appears that no apology was ever issued by members of the Bureau of Narcotics; the tone of their letters alone should have been reason enough for an expression of regret. It also appears that other persons and possibilities, such as Hjalmer Larson, were not investigated by state or by federal officials.

REFERENCES

13. Editorial. The Harrison law a national obligation. *Journal of the American Medical Association* 64:834, 1915.

14. Editorial. The physician and the Harrison Narcotic Law. *Journal of the American Medical Association* 64:834-835, 1915.

15. Queries and Minor Notes. Inquiries on the Harrison Antinarcotic Act. *Journal of the American Medical Association* 64:1265-1266, 1915.

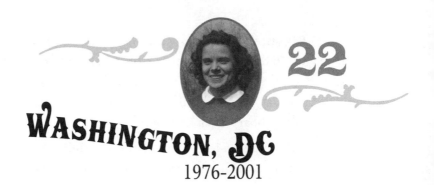

WASHINGTON, DC
1976-2001

Fran and I moved from Michigan to the Washington, DC, area in 1976, the U. S. bicentennial year. We lived there for 25 years, the longest we have remained in one place. Because our children were either in college or had completed school by that time, none of them moved with us. We were pleased that all of them were able to complete their higher educations. Rick has a degree from St. Olaf College and an M.D. degree from Michigan State University. Carol has a fine arts degree from MSU and an additional degree in nursing from California State University at Los Angeles. Alice's degrees, including a Ph.D. in physical chemistry, are from the University of Michigan. Our daughter-in-law, Cheryl, graduated in nursing from MSU. Carol's husband, Stuart, has a degree in engineering from the University of Michigan and a master's degree from the University of Southern California. Alice's husband, Ed, has a degree from the University of Wisconsin and a Ph.D. in physics from the University of Michigan.

THE NATIONAL INSTITUTES OF HEALTH

While Fran was helping to start the new Uniformed Services University of the Health Sciences (USUHS) in Bethesda, I spent my first year in the Washington area working in the Pediatric Oncology Branch (POB) of the National Cancer Institute (NCI), National Institutes of

Health (NIH), as a clinical associate. Also in my group were Gregory Reaman, Nili Ramu, and Lawrence Cohen. Larry later kindly cared for our grandchildren when they became sick while visiting us in Washington. After that year of training I took and passed the pediatric hematology/oncology board examination.

Among my supervisors in the POB were Philip A. Pizzo and David G. Poplack, who coauthored the wonderful book, *Principles and Practice of Pediatric Oncology*, the "bible" for pediatric oncologists. Both gentlemen were invariably kind and helpful. Phil became chair of the POB, and went on to become chair of pediatric hematology/oncology at Stanford University and dean of the Stanford medical school. David became chair of pediatric hematology/oncology at Baylor University in Houston, Texas.

Phil's special interest was infectious diseases. One of my patients was a young boy whose infection required treatment with penicillin. He was allergic to penicillin and had to be desensitized by the injection of miniscule doses of penicillin, with increases every 15 minutes until the proper dose was reached. Penicillin allergy and desensitization are very dangerous, with a risk of shock and even death, so that the physician must be ready with epinephrine at hand to counteract shock. Phil came down from his laboratory and chatted with me all afternoon throughout the procedure, which fortunately went well. I remember remarking to my patient, "Kerry, your mom is here, literally holding your hand, and Dr. Pizzo is here, figuratively holding mine!"

After my year as a clinical associate, I accepted an administrative position in the National Heart, Blood, and Lung Institute (NHLBI). Since I much preferred to be seeing patients, I left the NHLBI and accepted an offer from Howard University in the District of Columbia, where I eventually became a full professor of pediatrics and child health.

BONE MARROW TRANSPLANTATION

As a clinical associate at the NIH I had my second encounter with a bone marrow transplant patient. Allogeneic bone marrow transplantation is done by giving cells from the marrow of another person to a patient whose own marrow is not producing enough blood cells for the patient. My medical school classmate, Bob Good, is generally credited with performing the first successful bone marrow transplantation in 1968 with marrow from a donor.[16,17] The procedure is fraught with many possible problems, and major difficulties occur when the donor's cells attack the patient. This is called a graft-versus-host (GVH) reaction, and it can take many forms. When transplantation is used as part of cancer therapy, the patient is given such strong doses of anti-cancer drugs that the bone marrow, which is the source of the blood cells in the circulation, is essentially destroyed along with the cancer cells. This intense therapy is followed by allogeneic bone marrow transplantation, that is, replacement of the patient's bone marrow with bone marrow cells from a donor, or by autologous transplantation, that is, replacement with the patient's own cells that have been "harvested" earlier from the patient and preserved by super-freezing. Autologous bone marrow transplantation, which was not carried out in either of these two patients, is less dangerous.

I had seen my first allogeneic marrow transplant, in which the marrow from a sibling was given to a little boy with aplastic anemia, at Michigan State University. The patient's bone marrow was unable to produce enough blood cells for him to survive without frequent blood transfusions. He had a serious GVH reaction to the transplant procedure in the form of diarrhea that did not respond to any treatment and caused the lining of his upper and lower intestines essentially to be shed and eliminated.

My second transplant patient had been given an allogeneic bone marrow transplant as part of his cancer treatment at the NIH. This young man in his early twenties with a severe GVH from the bone marrow transplant was brought in one evening by his father. The patient's severe GVH reaction had caused his skin and the tissues of his joints to tighten up so that he was immobilized; he lay straightened out on a pallet, unable to move and barely able to speak. He had a urinary tract infection, but the young man decided, with the concurrence of his father, to refuse treatment.

It is important to recognize that since those early attempts, bone marrow transplantation has been immensely improved; the procedure is much safer, with fewer complications, and it can indeed be life-saving in the proper circumstances.

THE PEDIATRIC ONCOLOGY BRANCH

While at Howard University I was granted a year's sabbatical leave to work in the POB, and when I retired after ten years at Howard, I went back to the POB, this time as a guest researcher working with Dr. Ian T. Magrath on the problem of non-Hodgkin's lymphoma. My research project was a long term follow up study of Ian's non-Hodgkin's lymphoma patients; working with me on the project was June McCalla, a nurse practitioner in the POB.[18] Sometimes problems occur as a result of past treatment, while other difficulties can be related to having been severely ill. The NIH treatment protocols for non-Hodgkin's lymphoma had yielded very good cure rates, and most of the patients had adjusted to life after cancer and were living normal lives. Eventually, Ian moved to Belgium to further his work with the NCI, and I became an academic advisory member of the Long Term Follow Up Clinic staff of Children's National Medical Center (CNMC) in the District of Columbia. Follow-up by then had become recognized as extremely important for cured cancer patients, and it is now routine to keep track of cured cancer patients indefinitely.

AN INTERESTING PATIENT

One of the most interesting patients who came to the NIH for follow up was an airline pilot. He had been cured of his non-Hodgkin's lymphoma as a teenager, and he came in for his checkup as a long term survivor. He was an exceedingly attractive young man in his early thirties who had recently passed a rigorous physical examination by his own airline's physician that made him eligible for promotion and for piloting overseas flights. His only complaint, or rather, his wife's complaint, was infertility, and she was complaining bitterly. (In my opinion, he should have sent her home to her mother!) The couple was unable to conceive because he had been treated with cyclophospha- mide, a cancer chemotherapy drug that is known to cause sterility in males. He was reported to have had a normal electrocardiogram included in the airline physical examination. However, an echocardiogram per- formed by the NIH unfortunately turned out to be abnormal. This was, of course, a dilemma. Physician confidentiality precluded us from giv- ing this information to his airline physician, and as far as I know he is still a commercial pilot, making overseas flights for his airline.

LIVING IN THE WASHINGTON AREA

We lived at first in an apartment in Chevy Chase, Maryland, and later moved to a town house in Potomac, Maryland. Living in the Wash- ington, DC, area is very pleasant in many ways. There is very little cold weather although the seasons change, and spring in Washington lasts a long time, with a series of beautiful flowers being displayed—forsythia, dogwood, redbud, azaleas to start and from then on through autumn every type of blossom that can be imagined. We spent a great deal of time at the Smithsonian Institutes, admiring their superb collections, including botanical displays and the National Zoo—at no cost for admission to any of the exhibits. We visited the Viet Nam and Korean War monuments and the Franklin D. Roosevelt memorial, and we walked in Rock Creek Park and along the C and O Canal Towpath by the Potomac River. We were able to see many of the programs at the Kennedy Center. Because people like to visit our nation's capital, we had frequent visits from relatives and friends and could view the insti- tutes and monuments with guests on many occasions. A source of great pleasure to us was that Alice and Ed, with Deborah, moved to Greens- boro, North Carolina, a six hour trip away by automobile, and we could see them fairly often.

REFERENCES

16. Gatti, R. A., Meuwissen, H. J., Allen, H. D., Hong R., Good, R. A. Immunological reconstitution of sex-linked immunological deficiency. *Lancet* 1968;ii:1366-1369.

17. Good, R. A., Meuwissen, H. F., Hong, R., Gatti, R. A. Successful marrow transplantation for correction of immunological deficit in lymphopenic agammaglobulinemia and treatment of immunologically induced pancytopenia. *Exp Hematol* 1969;19:4-10.

18. Haddy, T. B., Adde, M. A., McCalla, J., *et al*. Late effects in long-term survivors of high-grade non-Hodgkin's lymphomas. *J Clin Oncol* 1998;16:2070-2079.

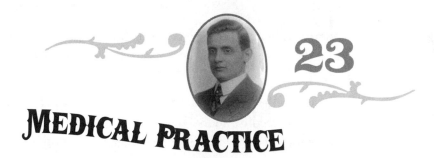

MEDICAL PRACTICE

THE LATER YEARS
1926-1940

he first sulfa drug came into general use in 1935. Although penicillin was discovered by the British scientist Fleming in 1928, the first clinical trials of the antibiotic were not carried out until 1941, in England. The first blood bank was established at Cook County Hospital, Chicago, in 1937. Dr. Robert E. Gross developed a method for ligating a patent ductus arteriosus at the Children's Hospital in Boston in 1938, and the following year Dr. Owen Wangensteen successfully performed the procedure on a child at the university hospital in Minneapolis.

My father had a number of colleagues to whom he turned for consultation. Patients who needed routine, uncomplicated operations such as appendectomies were sent in the early years either to New Ulm or to Marshall, but later almost exclusively to Dr. Frank Davis Gray at Marshall. Most patients with diagnostic problems, either medical or surgical, were referred to the Mayo Clinic. The Mayo Clinic charged according to the patient's ability to pay, and some paid very little. Charity patients went to the University of Minnesota Clinics and Hospitals. Veterans of the First World War, the Spanish-American War, and the Civil War were sent to the Veterans' Administration Hospital in Minneapolis. A few veterans of the Spanish-American War and the War Between the States were still living in Wabasso when I was a child. I particularly remember old Mr. Davis, who had been a drummer boy in the Civil War, participating in parades on Armistice Day (now called Veterans' Day).

One of my father's contacts at the Mayo Clinic was a fraternity brother and friend from medical school days, Dr. Charles Monte Piper. My brothers and sisters and I were delivered at home by my father, but on at least one occasion Dr. James Cosgriff came from Olivia to see my mother after a childbirth. I believe it was after my birth. (Dr. Cosgriff's son, James, was in my class in medical school.) Another fraternity brother and friend was Dr. Otto John Siefert of New Ulm. Once, when Ann, Ginger, and I were visiting our paternal grandparents in their retirement home in New Ulm, my grandmother became alarmed because Ginger was not eating very well. Dr. Siefert made a housecall at my father's request, and there were telephone calls back and forth. Eventually my parents were reassured that it was a simple case of homesickness.

MENTOR

My father looked upon Dr. Gray as a father figure or mentor. Henry A. Castle included a biographical sketch of Dr. Gray in his book, *Minnesota: Its Story and Biography, vols I-III*. (The Lewis Publishing Co., Chicago and New York, 1915). He frequently visited the Marshall Hospital, located approximately 30 miles west of Wabasso, and most likely assisted Dr. Frank Gray with surgical procedures on the patients he had referred. No doubt an informal exchange of information took place while conferring with Dr. Gray and other medical colleagues there.

CONTINUING MEDICAL EDUCATION

Keeping up with new medical and technological advances was, of course, extremely important to my father. Continuing medical education seminars and workshops were uncommon in those days, and if they had been available, Dr. Brey probably would not have felt comfortable taking the time to attend them. Working alone in Wabasso, without medical colleagues for convenient consultation, he must have felt professionally isolated. He kept in touch, however, with other physicians. He belonged to at least two medical organizations, the Minnesota State Medical Association [Figure 60] and the Southern Minnesota Medical Association [Figure 61], but meetings were held too far away for convenient, frequent attendance. He subscribed to *Minnesota Medicine*, published monthly by the Minnesota State Medical Association, and *The Journal-Lancet*, published twice monthly, which represented the medical profession for the states of Minnesota, North Dakota, South Dakota, and Montana, and was the official journal of the North Dakota and South Dakota State Medical Association.

MINNESOTA STATE MEDICAL ASSOCIATION
AND THE
REDWOOD-BROWN COUNTY Medical Society
DR. F. W. BREY
is a member in good standing to December 31st, 1939
Benjamin B. Souster — Sec'y Minn. Med. Assn.
Carl J. Fritsche — Sec'y. Med. Soc.

THIS IS TO CERTIFY THAT
Dr. F. W. Brey
Is a Member in Good Standing of the
Southern Minnesota Medical Association
And That He Has Paid His Dues in Full
to December 31, 1939
Secretary Southern Minnesota Medical Association

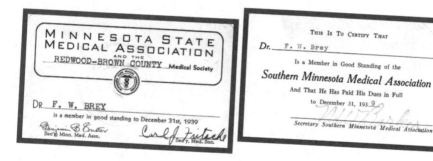

(From Left To Right)

Fig. 60: *Dr. Brey's 1939 membership card for the Minnesota State Medical Association. On the back of the card is a notification form to be submitted to the Medical Advisory Committee of the Association in case of a malpractice suit.*

Fig. 61: *Dr. Brey's 1939 membership card for the Southern Minnesota Medical Association.*

Several journals preserved among his records are noteworthy because they contained articles that were presumably of special interest to him. A copy of *The Journal-Lancet*, dated January 1, 1922, carries the following News Item: "Dr. Frank W. Brey, of Wabasso, was married last month to Miss Elizabeth Daub, of the same place. Dr. Brey was a 1910 graduate of the Medical School of the University of Minnesota." The November 1922 issue of the *New York Medical Journal and Medical Record: A Semimonthly Review of Medicine and Surgery* is titled the Genitourinary Number and is devoted to disorders of the urinary system and syphilis. *The Journal-Lancet* for December 1928 contains an article on toxemia of pregnancy and also a short paragraph advocating preventive immunization against diphtheria with toxin-antitoxin (three weekly injections of 1 ml each). Long term immunization against diphtheria was quite new at that time and represented an important step forward in the fight against the disease, since only short term immunization with antitoxin, in itself a valuable advance, had been available until then. Two copies of *Minnesota Medicine*, for January and May 1934 were probably of interest for their articles on the injection treatment of varicose veins and inguinal hernias.

Inside one of the journals is a three-page, blank, patient history and physical examination form from the office of New Ulm practitioner Dr. H. A. Vogel, suggesting that Dr. Brey was thinking of using a similar form in his own office.

Books were a major source of continuing medical education. Injection treatment appeared to have been fairly new, and was useful in treating hemorrhoids as well as varicose veins and inguinal hernias. His interest in the procedures, no doubt with the idea that they could be adapted for use in his office, is demonstrated by his preservation of two books that listed references for the injection treatment of hemorrhoids [Appendix D] and varicose veins [Appendix D]. A partial list of his textbooks, which are preserved in the library of my family home, is included in Appendix E. The list is incomplete because the newer and more valuable books were disposed of along with the office furniture and equipment when his practice was sold shortly before his death. The book on varicose veins by McPheeters is of interest because it is the only one in the collection written by a Minnesota physician. Dr. McPheeters was still practicing surgery in Minneapolis when I served my rotating internship at the Minneapolis General Hospital in 1947-1948. *The Diseases of Infancy and Childhood* by Holt used by my father was the seventh edition of the textbook; my class in pediatrics when I was in medical school (1943-1946) was assigned the eleventh edition of Holt's book (published, 1940).

Diseases of the Nose, Throat, and Ear contains a notation in the frontspiece written in my father's handwriting, "tonsil local, [page] 397." The page number refers to a colored plate of a pharynx with diseased tonsils; below the illustration is written, also in my father's handwriting, "Hypo ¼ gr (grain), morphin [sic] + 1/150 gr atropin [sic] 15 minutes before operation but immediately before novocain." Four pencilled-in lines, numbered consecutively, number one through four, show where the novocain injections were to be placed. Tonsillectomy was the surgical procedure that he most frequently performed. A local anesthetic was administered to adults prior to surgery, but children were put to sleep before the start of the procedure with the general anesthetic ether.

ADVERTISING

Placement of Dr. Brey's "business card" in the local *Wabasso Standard* constituted his professional advertising. He was no doubt included in the local telephone book, too. His "card" appeared, just below that of Dr. A. J. McLean, the dentist, in Arnold Bauer's book, *The Story of Wabasso*, in 1934. The City Drug Store, which my father no longer owned, was advertised on a different page.

"CENTRAL"

We had two telephones in our house, one hanging from the kitchen wall and the other in my parents' bedroom. They were box-like contraptions with a speaker in front and a lever on the right side of each box. When someone wanted to make a telephone call, he or she would crank the lever and ring the Wabasso telephone operator, who had an office with a switchboard downtown. She would answer, "Central," and proceed to place the call as instructed. A telephone line had been built through Wabasso in 1900 and a local exchange installed in 1902. For some years the exchange was located above the Citizens State Bank, but in 1919 the telephone system was completely overhauled and a new one-story building with basement was built for the exchange on Main Street.

One of the reasons why gossip got around so very quickly in Wabasso was because "Central" often entertained her friends in her office while continuing to operate the switchboard. Another reason was because, although we had a private line, all rural telephone lines were "party" lines. People on party lines were notified that someone was ringing them through a coded ring heard by every subscriber on the line—one ring or two, a short and long, or some other combination. In case of an emergency, Central would give the "general ring" that was recognized as a signal for all of the people on the line to answer their telephones. Individuals were not supposed to lift their receivers except for their own signals or a general ring, but of course everyone did.

Central took great pride in always knowing where "the doctor" was, so that she could reach him in case of an emergency, and in this way she functioned as an informal answering service. According to my mother, this was an entirely voluntary service on Central's part. That there were times when Central knew where her husband was, and she did not, was a continuing source of irritation to my mother.

News got around fast in Wabasso. My father had a patient whose abdominal distress was diagnosed as appendicitis. He telephoned Dr. Gray in Marshall, instructed the family to transport the patient to the Marshall Hospital, and went home to change his shirt before starting out himself on the drive to Marshall. Central hastened to be first with the news and called around to various friends, including one who happened to be our next-door neighbor. The neighbor excitedly informed my mother of the surgical emergency and stated that Dr. Brey was already on his way to Marshall with a patient who required an appendectomy. My mother received this bit of news over the garden fence just as my father, wearing a freshly laundered shirt, walked out of our front door toward his automobile.

EDUCATION

My father's commitment to the cause of education included the children of the community as well as his own children and young relatives. He took seriously his responsibilities as first a member, then later as the president, of the school board. (School board members were elected but were not paid for their efforts. As a result, not many people aspired to a place on the school board.) When new legislation to benefit the schools was being voted upon, inevitably unpopular because increased taxes would follow, he would often collect the "sick votes" during his travels around the countryside from those of his patients who could be depended upon to support the schools but were home-bound because of illness.

As the local health officer and school physician for the Wabasso Public Elementary and High Schools and for St. Anne's Elementary School, he supervised the medical aspects of the physical education programs. Arnold Gadow remembered, "In high school all of us had to go to see him. He would examine each [of us] before we played in sports. His office was a little building on Main Street [Figure 62]. A waiting room with a few chairs and then in the back is where he took us to be treated. A table to lie upon and all the instruments he used."

He carried out immunization programs for both schools, assembly-line fashion, with the students gathered in their gymnasiums. The scenes at several of them have remained vivid in my mind because,

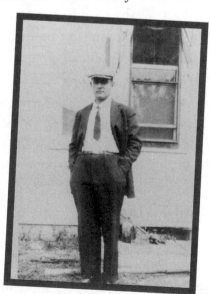

Fig. 62: *Frank W. Brey, M. D., outside his office, circa 1932 (from Haddy, R. I., et al.: The Journal of Family Practice 36:65-69, 1993).*

inevitably, one or more of the pupils would faint and have to be laid out, supine, on the floor. My siblings and I were never participants in these sessions. We were immunized at home, with my father using an approach he had developed after one or two sessions with six screaming children. The oldest, Ann, started to cry when she saw the needle; the other five quickly joined in; and bedlam ensued— all before any action had taken place. After those early experiences, he administered our injections after we were sound asleep in our beds. Nobody awakened, and a small start of surprise was the maximum reaction.

BANG'S DISEASE

Bang's disease, or contagious abortion in cattle, which is caused by the bacterium Brucella abortus, can cause brucellosis, or undulant fever, in human beings. Exposure results from drinking unpasteurized milk or from close contact with infected cows. Winford P. Larson and Julius P. Sedgwick, at the University of Minnesota, tested a large number of children with the antigen to Brucella abortus in 1913 and reported that 17% responded positively to the test, indicating that they had been exposed at some time to infected cows and that the infection was fairly widespread among Minnesota cattle herds. The first human cases of brucellosis in Minnesota were reported in 1929 by Frank J. Hirschblock. Later, the problem was studied in depth by Wesley Spink and his research team in the Department of Medicine at the University of Minnesota.

A cousin of mine had an early case of brucellosis, from the family's own cows, around the time when the disease was first being described. His father, my uncle, was obliged to get rid of the entire herd and avoid using the infected cattle yard for many years.

MENINGITIS

One of my father's first patients to receive an early sulfa drug was another cousin, and this must have taken place in the late 1930s because sulfa drugs did not become available until 1935. My father had made the diagnosis of spinal meningitis, a bacterial infection of the meninges, the membranes that cover the brain and spinal cord. No specific treatment was available at that time, and the disease was invariably fatal. He offered to try the new sulfa drug, which had just become available and was given by mouth. To everyone's surprise and gratification, my cousin recovered completely. His parents were warned, however, that their child would probably not do well in school. As it turned out, he did very well indeed, eventually becoming an executive with Northwest Airlines. In retrospect, he must have had meningococcal meningitis, caused by Neisseria meningitidis, a bacterium that responds to sulfa drugs. Sulfanilamide, the first sulfa drug to be available, was no doubt the drug that was used. This being one of the very early cases to be treated, the bacteria must have been exquisitely sensitive to the drug.

Although it was a potent drug, sulfanilamide is no longer in common use, but has been replaced by more effective and less toxic forms of sulfa, and by antibiotics. The sulfa group of anti-bacterial chemicals are not antibiotics but, rather, chemotherapeutic agents, or synthetically-produced compounds. The classification, antibiotics, is reserved for substances such as penicillin that are or were first produced by a microorganism (in the case of penicillin, by a strain of Penicillium fungi).

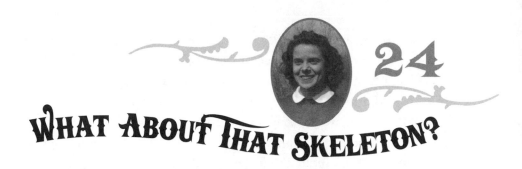

WHAT ABOUT THAT SKELETON?

My skeleton torso, which had been used to teach medical students how to do lumbar punctures, was stored upstairs in the garage of my family home, the Red House on the Hill in St. Paul. Hanging by its metal ring and still encased in its brown paper covering, it had been there since my family bought the property in 1946. When Fran and I started setting our affairs in order— we were by then living in Potomac, Maryland—we felt that we should include getting rid of any items, such as my skeleton, that might be embarrassing for someone else to explain sometime in the future. The skeleton would have to go.[19]

It soon became clear that getting rid of it would be far from simple, and we gave the matter a great deal of thought. We ruled out burning it because incinerating bones required a higher temperature than we could achieve in a bonfire or a stove, and we were reluctant to approach a crematorium with our problem. We ruled out burying it in the backyard because it might be dug up some day by a future owner, and suspicion might be directed at the previous owners of the property. Fran had a good idea. He said, "Give it back to the Department of Pharmacology at the University of Minnesota." Our daughter Alice, the physical chemist, had an even better idea. A friend of hers who was a professor of physical anthropology offered to use the bones for teaching her courses at her university.

Now we could consider the next phase of "Project Bones," which was: how to transport the skeleton. We ruled out the use of Federal Express and United Parcel Service. They always asked what was being shipped. So did the Post Office. When I telephoned my sister Ann and brother Paul, who were living in the family home, to let them know when I would be in St. Paul, we had not yet decided on a method of transportation. They replied that they would have everything ready for me.

"But shouldn't we invite Denise's children over for a last look?" inquired Ann. Our niece, Denise, had five children ranging at that time from four to fourteen years of age.

I said, "What? Invite the children?"

"Why, yes," said Ann. "They always look at the skeleton when they visit us. They often invite their friends to see it, too."

I said, "What? Invite their friends?"

"Why, yes," said Ann. "They all like to look at the skeleton."

"Absolutely not," I said, "Now I am sure that we must get rid of it!"

We set a date for my coming to St. Paul, and Ann went to the Post Office to ask where she could get a box made to order. She thought that a 48 x 12 x 14 inch box would be about the right size. "What will be in the box?" asked the postal assistant.

"A dress form," answered Ann, who is a retired home economist, "for a home economics class."

She stopped at a box store to order a pasteboard box made. "What will be in the box?" asked the clerk.

"A dress form," answered Ann, "for a home economics class."

When I arrived in St. Paul from half way across the U. S. continent, Paul had everything neatly laid out on an old strip of carpet in the garage. The skeleton was in pretty good shape except for several cracked ribs. The metal ring at the top and the wiring that held the vertebrae together were a little rusty. We stuffed the torso with newspapers, wrapped it in more newspapers, added several layers of cloth, and inserted it into the box. It fit perfectly.

"Wait," exclaimed Ann, "We can't send a box labeled 'Dress Form' to a Department of Anthropology!"

I said, "Let's send it to Alice." But sending a dress form to a Department of Chemistry didn't seem right either. So we sent the package to Alice at her home.

The same postal attendant was on duty when we brought the box to the Post Office. Fortunately, he already "knew" that the package contained a dress form, so he didn't ask what was in it.

A few days later we received a telephone call from Alice, reporting that the package had been duly delivered to its destination.

A post script: Our nephew Kyle was unhappy when he next visited the Red House on the Hill and found the skeleton gone. He cheered up considerably, however, after his Auntie Ann explained to him that the skeleton had come out of retirement and had gone to help teach anthropology students at Cousin Alice's university.

REFERENCE

19. Haddy, T. B. What about that skeleton in the garage? *The Pharos*, Alpha Omega Alpha Honor Medical Society, p 39, Autumn, 2001.

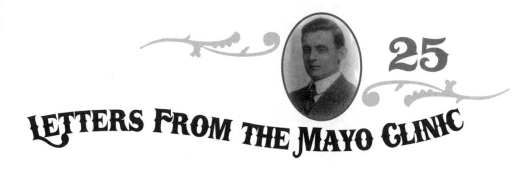

LETTERS FROM THE MAYO CLINIC

The Mayo Clinic was well established by the time Dr. Brey began practicing medicine. William Worrall Mayo had started his medical practice in Rochester, Minnesota, in 1863. He was joined by his sons, William James Mayo and Charles Horace Mayo, in the 1880s and subsequently by other physicians. The Mayo family practice developed into the prototype for private multispecialty group practice. The Mayo Clinic, founded in 1914, soon became a world famous referral center, respected for outstanding medical and surgical expertise and for its willingness to share information with visiting physicians. Dr. Brey was known to have referred patients to several other centers, including the University of Minnesota and the Veterans' Administration, but no reports from other referrals have been found.

The Mayo Clinic was a resource for obtaining help with difficult and puzzling medical problems, and physicians, at that time mostly from the Midwest, welcomed this assistance. The Mayo Clinic consultants routinely sent letters to referring physicians concerning their patients, with concise reports regarding the patients' evaluation and treatment as well as advice about follow-up care. The letters served to promote good relations with community physicians, and were also an important form of continuing medical education for the referring physicians.

A group of 113 original letters from Mayo Clinic physicians was found among Dr. Brey's medical records,[20] in a chest that had been in the breakfast room of the Red House since 1946. All of the letters were written between 1920 and 1929 except two, which were dated 1931 and 1935. The letters were arranged in alphabetic order according to patients' last names in a file labeled "Private Letters."

113 MAYO LETTERS

The 113 letters were written by 53 Mayo Clinic physicians, all of whom had MD degrees (Table 8). The letters concerned 81 patients, of whom 76 were seen in the clinic and five were not. Forty-nine patients were males, 29 were females, and the sex of three was not indicated. Eleven letters were about nine children, 94 were in regard to 67 adults, and eight letters concerned the five patients who had not been seen.

TABLE 8. *Characteristics of 76 patients referred to a major medical center by a rural Minnesota family practitioner in the 1920s and numbers of letters received for each category.*

	Males (n)	Females (n)	Sex not Indicated (n)	Total (n)	Letters (n)
Children	6	3	0	9	11
Adults	42	24	1	67	94
TOTAL	48	27	1	76	105

DESCRIPTION OF THE LETTERS

The letters were typewritten on high quality paper with a letterhead stating simply, "Mayo Clinic, Rochester, Minnesota." The name of the writer's section was added to most, but not all, of the letterheads. The letters were short, most of them less than a page in length. The date, the patient's clinic number, and the patient's name were invariably included, but, interestingly, the age and sex of the patient were never

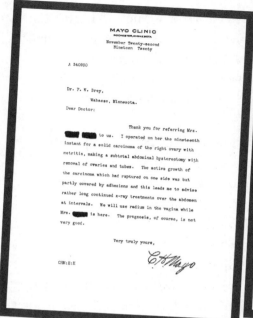

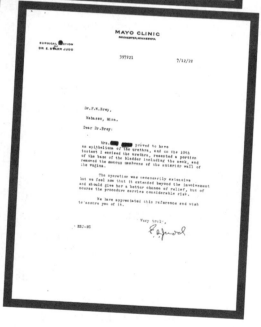

(Clockwise From Top Left)
Fig. 63: *Letter from Charles H. Mayo dated November 22, 1920, with report of major surgery for ovarian carcinoma.*

Fig. 64: *Letter from Henry S. Plummer dated October 6, 1921, stating that patient registered at the clinic, with promise to send report.*

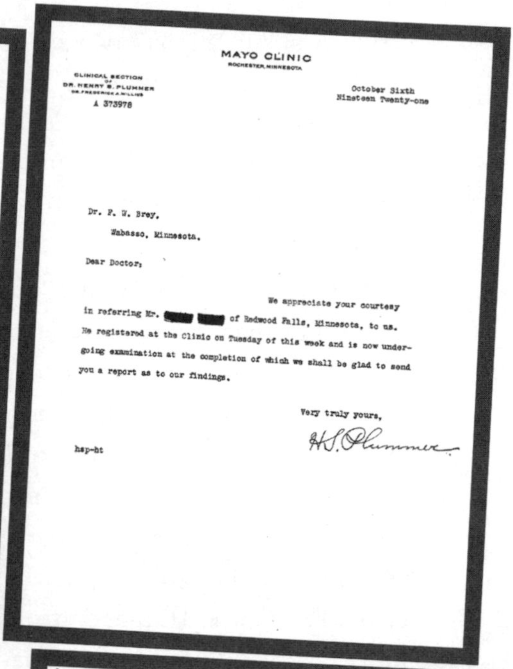

Fig. 65: *Letter from E. Starr Judd dated July 12, 1922, with report of major surgery for epithelioma of the urethra.*

mentioned. That the patient was a child could be deduced if he or she was referred to as a boy or girl, if there was mention of a parent, or if the letter originated in the Section of Pediatrics. For example, a patient referred to as "little [girl's name]," was clearly a female child. An adult patient's sex could be similarly deduced. Mr. before a name indicated that the patient was a man. A married woman was designated Mrs., followed by her husband's first name, never her own, and her husband's last name. An unmarried woman was called Miss, followed by her first and last names.

The letters were invariably gracious and usually began with an expression of thanks for the referral. Although brief and to the point, they contained all essential information. Seven writers mentioned that the patient was introduced by a letter or note from Dr. Brey, but it seems likely that most of his referrals were accomplished by telephone, with perhaps a few patients being self-referred. One letter each was written by Charles H. Mayo (Figure 63), Henry S. Plummer (Figure 64), and E. Starr Judd (Figure 65). Although there were two additional letters from Dr. Charles H. Mayo, his name was followed in both instances by an "E", probably indicating that they had been signed by a secretary. Dr. C. H. Mayo was mentioned twice and Dr. E. Starr Judd once by other physicians as having been called in to consult on difficult surgical cases. Four letters written by Dr. P. S. Hench were notable for their detail, and two of Dr. Hench's letters contained an additional single-spaced sheet filled with comprehensive information about arthritis and instructions for its treatment.

The largest number of letters, eight, was written by Dr. Dorr F. Hallenbeck. An interesting letter from Dr. Monte C. Piper, Dr. Brey's medical school classmate and fraternity brother, one of five letters written by him, expressed his appreciation of "your kind entertainment while we were there," saying "we enjoyed our hunt with you." Only one letter was signed by a woman, Leda June Stacy, from the Clinical Section of Dr. Leda June Stacy and Dr. Della G. Dripps. There was a 114th Mayo letter, the single letter in Dr. Brey's file that was not from a physician. Anna Edmonson, general secretary, from the Division of Correspondence, wrote, "Thank you for referring [patient's name]. He registered at the Clinic this morning and is undergoing examination.... We shall be glad to do whatever we can for this patient and send you a report of our findings later."

DIAGNOSIS AND TREATMENT

Patient characteristics of the 76 patients who were seen in consultation are listed in Table 8. Eleven letters concerned nine children [Table 9], all of whom were reported to have a single primary diagnosis. Two had residual poliomyelitis, and three had unusually severe fractures. Other miscellaneous problems, one each, included post-influenzal encephalitis, acute gastroenteritis, hemangioma, and no definite diagnosis.

The primary diagnoses for 67 adult patients, about whom 94 letters were written, are listed in Table 10. Thirty had a single primary diagnosis, while 37 had up to four additional secondary diagnoses listed. The most common primary diagnoses were neurosis and no definite diagnosis (including one fever of unknown origin), with appendicitis being the third most common primary diagnosis. The 67 adult patients had 76 secondary diagnoses, which are listed in Table 11. The most common secondary diagnoses were infected teeth and infected tonsils, with neurosis being the third most frequent secondary diagnosis.

Twenty-two operations were performed [Table 12], most commonly for general surgical problems, followed by cancer and infection. Of 38 patients who were considered to have surgical situations, 16 were not operated upon. One patient with "subsiding" appendicitis had an appendectomy; however, three patients with "subacute," "chronic," and ruptured appendixes were followed with observation. A rectal fissure was treated with warm irrigations. Three patients had kidney stones; one passed after cystoscopic manipulations, one passed spontaneously, and the third patient was advised that the stone should pass. Two patients with stomach carcinoma were diagnosed without surgical intervention and palliative treatment was advised. A patient with hepatic carcinoma had exploratory surgery, but no tissue was removed. Of the nine patients with infected tonsils, only three had tonsillectomies, the other six most likely being sent home to have their operations performed there.

Eleven patients received a diagnosis of neurosis, referred to as "nerves," anxiety, or chronic nervous exhaustion, of whom several also had an element of depression or recurrent depression. Recommended treatment included bromids [sic] and a change of scenery (California was mentioned in one instance).

The correspondence about five patients who were not seen [Table 13] concerned a high urine sugar for two, confirmed or reiterated previous instructions for two, and requested the address of the fifth patient.

The 113 letters from Mayo Clinic physicians, with reports concerning patients who had been referred, were probably a unique service for that time. They reveal a picture of serious medical problems faced by family practitioners in the early twentieth century. The referring physicians, many of them from the Midwest, were kept informed of their patients' treatment and progress. They could feel confident that their patients were given up-to-date treatment, and they were further advised about appropriate follow up care. The letters, brief as they were, played an extremely important role in maintaining good relations with community physicians. They also served as a form of continuing medical education for family physicians, who often practiced in isolated areas and whose access to new medical knowledge was limited.

It is not surprising that the most common referrals were for surgical problems, followed closely by cancer and infection, since rural areas lacked the facilities and personnel required to perform complex surgery. Nor is it surprising that severe neurosis was a frequent primary and secondary diagnosis. It could be argued that neurosis complicated the diagnostic thinking of the referring physician, but most likely the primary care physician's aim in seeking a second opinion was to reassure the neurotic patient. No obstetric cases, mental illnesses other than depression, or sexually transmitted diseases were reported. No doubt the 150 mile distance from Wabasso to Rochester precluded travel for obstetric patients at critical times when help was most needed. Patients with severe mental disorders were not referred to the Mayo Clinic because at that time most patients with mental disorders were hospitalized in the nearby Rochester State Hospital. Although none of the 113 letters mentioned what were then called venereal diseases, that is, diseases transmitted by sexual contact, Dr. Brey frequently referred patients with sexually transmitted diseases (STDs) to the Mayo Clinic.

TABLE 9. *Primary and secondary diagnoses reported for 9 child patients referred to a major medical center by a rural Minnesota family practitioner in the 1920s.*

Primary Diagnosis	Complications and/or Secondary Diagnoses	Patients (n)
Fracture		3
Humerus		
Skull	Extradural hemorrhage	
Skull	Jacksonian seizures	
Poliomyelitis, residual		2
	Disability leg & shoulder Equinovarus & talipes valgus, atrophy lower extremities, underdeveloped, undernourished, migraine headaches	
Encephalitis, post-influenzal	Sleep disturbance, behavior disturbance, respiratory syndrome	1
Acute gastroenteritis	Dehydration, perforated ear drum, gingivitis	1
Haemangioma [sic]		1
No definite diagnosis	Fever, rigidity of arms	1
TOTAL		9

TABLE 10. *Primary diagnoses reported for 67 adult patients referred to a major medical center by a rural Minnesota family practitioner in the 1920s.*

Primary Diagnosis	Number	Percent
Neurosis	6	8.9
No definite diagnosis 5/fever of unknown origin 1	6	8.9
Appendicitis 4/acute abdomen 1	5	7.5
Angina pectoris 1/mitral stenosis 1/myocardial degeneration 1	3	4.4
Kidney stone	3	4.4
Cystic mastitis with fibroadenoma of breast	3	4.4
Stomach cancer	2	3.0
Ulcer, gastric 1/duodenal 1	2	3.0
Hemorrhoids 1/rectal fistula 1	2	3.0
Epigastric pain 1/cardiac (stomach) spasm 1	2	3.0
Maxillary antrum infection	2	3.0
Arteriosclerosis	2	3.0
Diabetes	2	3.0
Arthritis, infectious 1/gouty 1	2	3.0
Vaginal bleeding	2	3.0
Acute pelvic inflammation	1	1.5
Ovarian cancer	1	1.5
Breast cancer	1	1.5
Liver carcinoma	1	1.5
Urethral epithelioma	1	1.5
Hypernephroma	1	1.5
Squamous cell epithelioma	1	1.5
Factitious ulcer	1	1.5
Phlegmon (cellulitis)	1	1.5
Abscess of neck	1	1.5
Tuberculosis	1	1.5
Asthma	1	1.5
Inguinal hernia	1	1.5
Epididymitis	1	1.5
Pyelonephritis	1	1.5
Biliary cirrhosis	1	1.5
Middle ear infection	1	1.5
Tinnitis	1	1.5
Trifacial neuralgia	1	1.5
Pernicious anemia	1	1.5
Corneal ulcer	1	1.5
Spina bifida	1	1.5
Fracture, compound, comminuted	1	1.5
TOTAL	67	100

TABLE 11. *Secondary diagnoses reported for 67 adult patients referred to a major medical center by a rural Minnesota family practitioner in the 1920s.*

Secondary Diagnoses	Number	Percent
Septic teeth, tooth abscess, pyorrhea	14	18.2
Tonsillitis, septic tonsils, fibrous tonsils, tonsillar abscess	9	11.6
Neurosis	5	6.5
Cholecystitis	4	5.2
Prostatitis, enlarged prostate	4	5.2
Tuberculosis	2	2.6
Constipation	2	2.6
Hemorrhoids	2	2.6
Deafness, poor hearing	2	2.6
Arteriosclerosis, forgetfulness	2	2.6
Enlarged thyroid/goiter	2	2.6
Bronchitis	2	2.6
Hemoptysis	1	1.3
Pleurisy	1	1.3
Severe anemia	1	1.3
Retroverted uterus	1	1.3
Metritis (inflammation of the uterus)	1	1.3
Seborrheic dermatitis	1	1.3
Sulfur dermatitis	1	1.3
Leukoplakia	1	1.3
Basal cell carcinoma	1	1.3
Infected dermoid cyst	1	1.3
Hydronephrosis	1	1.3
Hematuria	1	1.3
Cystitis	1	1.3
Pyuria	1	1.3
Myositis	1	1.3
Arthritis	1	1.3
Spondylitis	1	1.3
Hernia	1	1.3
Failing heart	1	1.3
Hypertension	1	1.3
Stomach complaints	1	1.3
Tophi both ears (uric acid crystals)	1	1.3
Mastoiditis	1	1.3
Hemiplegia	1	1.3
Trophic ulcers	1	1.3
Dislocation of hips, bilateral	1	1.3
TOTAL	76	100

TABLE 12. *Twenty-two surgical procedures performed in 22 of 67 adult patients referred to a major medical center by a rural Minnesota family practitioner in the 1920s.*

Nature of Problem	Surgical Procedure (n)	No Surgery (n)	Patients in Category (n)
Surgical problem (24)			
Tonsillitis	3	6	9
Appendicitis	1	3	4
Cholecystitis[1]	1	3	4
Cystic mastitis/fibroadenoma[1]	3	0	3
Acute abdomen	1	0	1
Hemorrhoids	1	0	1
Rectal fistula	0	1	1
Inguinal hernia, bilateral	1	0	1
Cancer (9)			
Stomach	0	2	2
Breast	1	0	1
Liver[2]	1	0	1
Ovary	1	0	1
Hypernephroma	1	0	1
Urethral epithelioma	1	0	1
Squamous epithelioma	1	0	1
Basal cell carcinoma	0	1	1
Infection (5)			
Abscess drained	2	0	2
Maxillary sinus antrum	2	0	2
Myringotomy	1	0	1
	22	16	38

1   One patient had two procedures, a cholecystectomy and a breast amputation.

2   The patient with carcinoma of the liver had an abdominal exploration but no tissue biopsy was obtained.

TABLE 13. *Eight Mayo Clinic letters were in reference to five patients not seen or not seen at that time.**

Subject of Letter	Diagnosis	Treatment	Number of Patients
Report on urine specimen, patients not seen	Diabetes mellitis	Not stated	2
Clarifying or reiterating previous instructions for patients seen previously	Not stated	1) Cooley's mixed toxins 2) Potassium iodid [sic], Fowler's solution	2
Request for patient's address, patient seen previously	Not stated	Not stated	1

*One male, two females, two sex not designated.

Records pertaining to their cases were kept locked in his office safe and were destroyed by my mother after his death.

Medical practice today differs from practice in the nineteen twenties in a number of ways. Child abuse was a concept that was not well known in the 1920s. Could any of the three children who were treated for serious fractures have been the victims of abuse? Currently, this possibility would be considered in the differential diagnosis, and an evaluation by social services might be requested.

Today's patients with infectious diseases, insulin-dependent diabetes, and many forms of cancer can be treated effectively with antibiotics, insulin, and chemotherapeutic agents, respectively. The introduction of various cardiovascular medications, angiography, and cardiac surgery has remarkably improved the treatment of atherosclerotic coronary heart disease. The advent of histamine H_2-receptor antagonists and proton pump inhibitors has revolutionized the treatment of peptic ulcer disease. Anxiety and depression are now more effectively managed with advances in psychotherapeutic techniques and the introduction of medications such as the tricyclic antidepressants and selective seritonin reuptake inhibitors. Cortisone and its derivatives can be used to treat arthritic and various autoimmune disorders.

Some very basic general principles have not changed. For example, Mayo Clinic surgeons often chose a judicious course of observation for general surgical as well as for urologic and gynecologic problems, rather than immediately operating. On the other hand, major operations, such as hysterectomy with bilateral oophorectomy for ovarian carcinoma, are still the accepted initial treatments for some cancers.

REFERENCE

20. Haddy, R. I., Haddy, T. B. 113 Letters from the Mayo Clinic: a Pattern of Medical Referrals in the Early 20th Century. *Mayo Clinic Proceedings* 77:213-215, 2002.

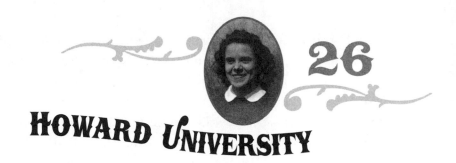

HOWARD UNIVERSITY

oward University in the District of Columbia is one of the two
historically black schools of higher education in the United
States that has a medical school. It was founded after the Civil
War for the higher education of freed slaves by a general who had fought
in the Union Army. I was attracted when I received an offer to teach in
the Howard University Department of Pediatrics and Child Health. The
current pediatric hematologist/oncologist, the only black one in the U. S.,
had moved to Meharry University. There were several reasons for my
interest. First, I had been doing purely administrative work at the
National Heart, Lung and Blood Institute; as an associate professor at
Howard University, I would have the opportunity to see patients and
teach. Second, Dr. Melvin E. Jenkins, chair of the department, was obviously a man of great integrity who was devoted to academic excellence.
Dr. John Downing, who became the next chair upon Dr. Jenkins' retirement, was also a man of great integrity although not quite so strongly
inclined toward academics. My respect and admiration for both of them
has continued through the years. Third, since black children are less
likely than white children to develop cancer, I thought there would be
an opportunity for me to make a contribution to medicine by investigating this interesting clinical group.

So I came to work in an institution in which I was again a minority—as a woman in medicine I had been a minority ever since entering

medical school. By this time women were being well accepted in the medical field, but being white in a black institution introduced another issue for me to deal with. For the first time, I had a partner, Dr. Sohail R. Rana. He and I continued to interact with the medical hematology and oncology specialists, Drs. Oswaldo Castro and Elliott Perlin, both of whom were extremely knowledgeable and cooperative. Dr. Rana, who was originally from Pakistan, had received exemplary training there and in the United States, and with his expertise and compassionate care of patients he soon became a model for the medical students and residents.

RESENTMENT

The black staff members at Howard were pretty much like people everywhere; a few were biased against me because of my race, but many if not most seemed to go out of their way to be kind. Unfortunately, among those who were clearly biased were a couple of young women pediatricians who had large chips on their shoulders. There had been another such young woman in the Department of Medicine at Michigan State University. These women were not helpful in promoting the aims of their departments because they made life unpleasant for non-black faculty members. As far as the patients were concerned, I had never felt any bias in the past from any patients because of being a woman, and I felt no bias among the patients at Howard because of my sex or my race.

DRIVING TO WORK IN THE DISTRICT

Howard University is located in a high crime section of the District of Columbia, and my teaching obligations included additional travel to the DC General Hospital in another section of the District, as well as to Greater Southeast Hospital in Anacostia, both hospitals located in even higher crime areas than Howard University Hospital. Although the hospitals were perfectly safe inside, driving to and from them required some thought. My car was a very small, neutral-colored Plymouth sedan, which I drove sedately, with the intent of not calling attention to myself in any way. I was fortunate in rarely having to go in at night, so my driving was mostly during daylight hours. On the few occasions when it was necessary for me to go to the hospital at night, I tried to keep the car moving at all times, attempting to time my arrival at intersections when the lights were green so that I would not have to stop. If the lights were red and no cars were coming from any direction, I kept going and drove right on through the intersection in spite of the red lights. I was careful to keep the doors locked. Sometimes, when I had forgotten, people driving alongside me honked and motioned to me to press down the lock button. Interestingly, on two occasions, when I stopped to ask directions in Anacostia, an even more dangerous area than the District itself, the persons I spoke to immediately got into their automobiles and led me to Greater Southeast Hospital.

CHILDREN WITH AIDS

I first saw children with acquired immunodeficiency syndrome (AIDS) at Howard University Hospital. The first patient was an infant under one year of age from the West Indian Island of Tobago. Dr. Jenkins had been lecturing there, and the infant, whose parents came from East India, was presented to him with a puzzling group of bacterial and viral infections, including iritis, an infection of the iris of the eyes, which I had never seen before. Dr. Jenkins had invited the parents to bring their child to Howard University for diagnosis and treatment. Children with AIDS have very different symptoms and signs from adults with AIDS, and at that time childhood AIDS had not been well described. On the basis of the multiple infections displayed by the child, we made the presumptive diagnosis, which was confirmed when the human immunodeficiency virus (HIV) was grown in the public health laboratory.

The other child was a pretty little 18-month-old girl who was known to be positive for HIV. This toddler had been born to an infected mother, but she so far showed no external signs of disease and appeared well. Her mother had been in prison for the first year and one-half of the child's life, so she lived on the pediatric wards, with the nurses giving her a great deal of attention. After the mother was discharged from jail, she took her child home and brought her to the hospital for weekly check-ups. The mother was troublesome in the pediatric outpatient clinic. She had been known to steal from the resident physicians' lockers, and the social workers were wary of her because she asked them for boxes of diapers for the child and then sold the diapers on the street for drug money.

My experience with the mother and child was one I would not like to repeat. After I finished giving the child her regular check-up one day in clinic, the mother asked me if I would replace the child's little gold earrings. On her previous visit the earrings had been removed because they were screwed too tightly, and the mother had been advised to leave them off for awhile. I said, "No." Then she asked me if I would hold the child while she put them in. I reluctantly said, "OK," but I had failed to note that the mother was high on drugs. When she tried to insert the poles of the earrings, her hands were shaking so badly that she missed the pierced holes and caused bleeding. I stopped the process immediately, but there was a lot of blood around and it took me awhile to clean up. The mother's comment, repeated several times throughout the entire procedure: "Too bad, doctor, that you don't know what you're doing!" Interestingly, when I emerged from the examining room after everything was over, I found all of the clinic nurses standing outside the door, looking concerned. Not one of them had come in to help. Even though I had worn gloves throughout the entire procedure, I worried until I was tested and proved negative for HIV some months later.

FAILED TO JOIN AN NIH STUDY GROUP

Because the number of childhood cancer patients never increased enough to enable Howard University to join one of the national clinical cancer study groups, my associate and I were limited in the amount of clinical research we could perform. I later learned that most of the District's black childhood cancer patients were cared for at Children's National Medical Center. Dr. Rana went on to make a name for himself working with AIDS children.

LOOKING BACK ON TEN YEARS

I have warm memories my ten years at Howard University, of many good friends and valuable experiences. However, my time there confirmed what I have always believed: any institution that is founded for or has as its special purpose the interests of a religious, ethnic, or racial group, or even a certain social class (I know of two medical schools that prefer to have their medical staff belong to the upper social classes) is handicapped in achieving true excellence. The only attribute to be considered should be merit.

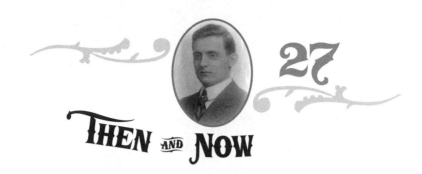

THEN AND NOW

The discovery of the bacillus Corynebacterium diphtheriae and the role of its toxin in the 1880s had opened the way for the production of an antitoxin for the treatment of diphtheria in 1895. In 1924, clinical trials of diphtheria toxoid for the prevention of diphtheria took place in New York. Louis S. Sauer developed the current vaccine for pertussis (whooping cough) at Northwestern University, and immunization against pertussis began in the early to mid-1930s. Because tetanus (lockjaw) was rare in western nations, tetanus toxoid was not widely used until the Second World War. Its effectiveness in the uniformed services of England and the United States led to its inclusion in infant immunization schedules.

Patients sometimes wonder, nowadays, what medical care was like in the kinder, gentler, "olden days." Physicians wonder, too. While he was at Wright State University in Dayton, Ohio, our son, Richard Ian Haddy, M. D., who is a professor of family medicine, studied my father's office records and identified some major differences between family practice a half-century ago and today. He and his colleagues compared the diagnoses from Dr. Brey's mid-1930s billing records, which had been preserved by my sister, Ann C. Brey, with diagnoses from a modern rural group practice in Yellow Springs, Ohio. They published their findings in The Journal of Family Practice in 1993.[21]

TABLE 14. *List of 244 diagnoses and procedures from Dr. Brey's day books, dated June 6, 1934, through September 25, 1935, compiled by Richard I. Haddy, M. D. and colleagues.*[21]

Diagnoses/Procedures	Number
Abscess, incision and drainage, follow-up	26
Immunization ("vaccination"), diphtheria	24
Mastoiditis, post-drainage, follow-up	17
Epididymitis, scrotal tap	14
Otitis media, post myringotomy, follow-up	14
Tonsillectomy and adenoidectomy	14
Arthritis ("Rheumatism"), follow-up	11
Abscess, incision and drainage	8
Fracture, major bone, follow-up	7
Pneumonia, follow-up	6
Pertussis (Whooping cough)	5
Uterine prolapse, pessary placement, follow-up	5
Abortion (Miscarriage), spontaneous, follow-up	4
Counseling	4
Measles, hemorrhagic, with pneumonia, follow-up	4
Physical examination, infant (Well baby check)	4
Renal colic ("Kidney stone"), follow-up	4
Birth, vaginal	3
Lymphangitis ("Blood poisoning"), leg, follow-up	3
Pneumonia	3
Otitis media, myringotomy	3
Abscess/infection	2
Asthmatic bronchitis, follow-up	2
Birth, Cesarean	2
Eczema	2
Eye glasses	2
Fracture, major bone	2
Laceration, repair	2
Lumbar strain ("Lumbago"), follow-up	2
Puncture wound, follow-up	2
Urethritis, follow-up	2
Vaginitis, follow-up	2
Abortion, threatened	1
Adenitis	1
Arthritis ("Rheumatism")	1
"Colitis," descending colon	1
Dermatitis, candidal ("Diaper rash")	1

TABLE 14. *Cont.*

Diagnoses/Procedures	Number
Diphtheria	1
Diphtheria, antitoxin administration	1
Diphtheria, follow-up	1
Hemorrhoids, external ("Piles")	1
Impetigo	1
Influenza	1
Lumbar radiculopathy ("Sciatic rheumatism")	1
Lymphangitis ("Blood poisoning"), leg	1
Mastitis, infant	1
Measles, hemorrhagic, with pneumonia	1
Otitis media	1
Pertussis ("Whooping cough")	1
Physical examination	1
Puncture wound	1
Renal colic ("Kidney stone")	1
Rhinitis, seasonal ("Hay fever")	1
Seizures, infantile	1
Sprain, ankle	1
Tonsillitis	1
Urethritis	1
Uterine prolapse, pessary placement	1
Vaginitis	1
Vision loss	1
Varicose veins, sclerosing	1
Varicose veins, follow-up	1

<u>Patient Age</u>

Infant	16
Child	97
Adult	131

<u>Patient Gender</u>

Male	140
Female	89
Infant, unrecorded	15

<u>Site of Encounter</u>

Office	148
Housecall	62
Country call	34

THE 1930s

Dr. Brey's billing records were available for the period between June, 1934, and September, 1935. Of 244 diagnoses or procedures listed (Table 14), the most common were related to infections, surgical or other procedures, and their follow-up. Most frequent was the incision and drainage of an abscess (26 cases). Diphtheria immunization, which had recently become available, was the second most frequent procedure (24 cases). In third place was incision and drainage of the mastoid, a bone located immediately behind the ear, for infection caused by advanced or chronic ear infection (17 cases). These were followed, fourth, by incision and drainage of the ear drum for acute infection of the middle ear (14 cases), and, fifth, incision and drainage of the scrotum for excess fluid (14 scrotal taps). The latter procedures were all performed upon the same patient, probably as a result of chronic gonorrhea. Sixth on the list was tonsillectomy and adenoidectomy, usually carried out because of recurrent throat infections (14 cases). Specific information about venereal diseases, now referred to as sexually transmitted diseases (STDs), was not found. These records, which had been stored in my father's office safe, were destroyed by my mother upon his death.

The rural Ohio group listed 286 diagnoses for the three months between April and June, 1989, with none of the top five involving surgical procedures. Most frequent was upper respiratory tract infection, including the common cold (13 cases); followed by hypertension (high blood pressure) (12 cases); hyperlipidemia (elevated blood lipids) (11 cases); adult history and physical examination (10 cases); and allergic rhinitis (hay fever) (9 cases). Only nevus (skin lesion) removal, which tied for fifth place (9 cases), involved a surgical procedure.

COMPARISON TO 1989

None of Dr. Brey's most common diagnoses appeared among the modern diagnoses listed by the Yellow Springs group, probably because the easy availability of antibiotics had eliminated them. Notably absent from his records were hypertension, hyperlipidemia, and depressive/

anxiety disorders. Although not recognized in the early twentieth century, these are among the most common disorders seen by present-day family physicians. It is questionable whether blood pressure was routinely measured in the early days, and the risk from elevation of the blood pressure may not have been well understood. In any case, there was no specific medication that could be prescribed for lowering high blood pressure. In the rural Ohio practice, patients were seen for depression or its follow-up (6 cases). Dr. Brey's list contained office counseling, unspecified (4 cases), which may well have been for depression or anxiety. The authors point out differences, not only in the day-to-day practice of the family physicians, but also in the way patients perceived illness. People did not see their physicians for common colds, tension headaches, allergic rhinitis, or routine adult check-ups, as they do today. Dr. Brey listed four infant check-ups, while the Yellow Springs practice had none, no doubt because children in their area were being seen by pediatricians. Other interesting diagnoses seen in the Wabasso practice but not in the Ohio practice were pneumonia (6 cases), whooping cough (5 cases), and hemorrhagic measles with pneumonia (4 cases). Five patients with uterine prolapse required pessary placement; today this condition would have been alleviated with a surgical procedure.

DR. BREY'S TRANSPORTATION AND FEES

Visits to his office, where he also performed minor surgery, made up sixty percent of Dr. Brey's patient encounters. The other forty percent were house calls and country calls. In the 1930s his transportation was by automobile, with a Model T or Model A Ford, except when roads became impassable from snow. The fee for an office visit was $2.00, one-tenth of the $20.00 fee charged for an office visit in the Ohio practice. The fee for a housecall was $3.00, plus an additional one dollar for each mile traveled in the country. Distances traveled to farm homes were usually between one and ten miles. No housecalls were made by the modern group. Dr. Brey charged $25.00 for a tonsillectomy and adenoidectomy, $30.00 for an obstetrical delivery (referred to as a "confinement"), and $35.00 for reducing and immobilizing a major fracture. Of special interest were two Cesarean births, evidently performed on a kitchen table in the home, for a fee of $35.00 each. That this actually happened is a difficult for us to understand today, but other physicians from early times, who had no one but themselves to rely upon, have reported performing surgical procedures on kitchen tables.

Dr. Brey rarely sent out bills and his collection rate was not known, although it must have been very low, perhaps ten to twenty percent at the height of the depression. At his death, over $100,000 remained on the books, uncollected.

THE CURRENT ROLE OF FAMILY PRACTICE?

At present, only one-third of active physicians in the United States are primary physicians, compared to fifty to seventy percent of those in other developed countries. Primary physicians include those in family practice, general pediatrics, and internal medicine. A number of developments improved the status of family physicians. The American Medical Association Section on General Practice was established in 1946, the American Academy of Family Practice followed in 1947, and family practice became a specialty with a three-year residency requirement and its own board certification in 1969. In spite of these efforts and the perceived need, however, fifteen percent or fewer of physicians graduating today plan to practice general medicine.

Ironically, the famous Flexner report of 1910, which contributed so heavily to the excellence of American medicine, appears to have also assisted in the decline of family practice.[21] As a result of Abraham Flexner's report, most of the deficient medical schools, and there were many, closed. The ones who remained open made great efforts to improve; and along with improvement came increased emphasis upon research, followed by the establishment of medical specialties and their individual boards. Physicians who specialized tend to receive greater respect and higher incomes. Not surprisingly, there has been a shift toward specialization and sub-specialization among young physicians in training and a gradual decrease in the number who entered the practice of general medicine.

Other ideas for health care to the underserved can be considered. The Mayo Clinic, for example, has implemented an innovative solution to the shortage of rural health care, with its successful network of clinics in rural southern Minnesota as well as in parts of Iowa and Wisconsin. Clinics attended by nurse practitioners or physician assistants are held daily or several times each week in most of the clinics, with a physician coming once or twice weekly to see the problem cases.

NOT ENOUGH DOCTORS?

In actuality, the United States appears to be facing not only a shortage of primary practitioners, but an overall shortage of physicians. Medical school applications have fallen by 30% since 1996. When I applied for medical school, there were ten or eleven applicants for every place, but today there are only two applicants for every place in medical school classes. Almost 40% of the physicians in practice today are 50 years of age or older. It appears that studying either law or business is more appealing to students of higher education. Reasons for the lack of interest in medicine as a career include the long training period before an income can be earned; the long working hours, both during training and after completing training; and the fact that physicians' incomes, except for those practicing a few selected specialties, are not particularly high. An additional deterrent might be the malpractice threat. Legal action against a physician occurs infrequently, but it is devastating to the person who is sued when it happens.

REFERENCES

21. Haddy, R. I., Hill, J. M., Costarella, B. R., Gordon, R. E., Adegbile, G. S. A., Van Niman, C. M., Markert, R. J. A comparison of rural family practice in the 1930s and today. *The Journal of Family Practice* 36:65-69, 1993.

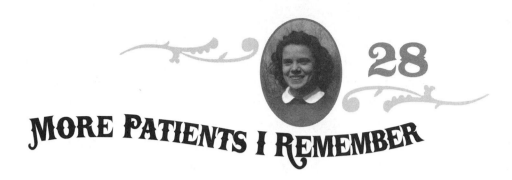

MORE PATIENTS I REMEMBER

When the entire health care team has done its best for a patient and the treatment is not successful, those are indeed discouraging times. Even more discouraging, however, is the situation when an effective treatment is available and the child's parents refuse treatment. An important aspect of good health care is knowing when and where to turn for help in such difficult situations.

PARENTS WHO REFUSE MEDICAL CARE FOR THEIR CHILDREN

A two-year-old boy known to have hemophilia was brought in to the Howard University Hospital because his parents could not stop his bleeding. This little boy had been playing on the floor with a knife and had accidentally cut his tongue. After a few days of oozing, his hemoglobin had dropped to the point where he was anemic. Hemophilia is characterized by a deficiency of clotting factor VIII. The disorder is passed from mother, who is not affected, to son. When bleeding occurs, it does not stop on its own, and effective treatment with the intravenous injection of factor VIII, either as fresh frozen plasma or a cryoprecipitate of plasma is required. The mother was a Jehovah's Witness, a member of a religious group who eschew therapy with blood products of any kind, and she refused treatment.

We held a meeting of several faculty persons, including my chairman, the child abuse specialist, the attending physician on the ward, and myself, to decide what to do. Dr. Jenkins and I, who were the senior physicians present, wanted to go to court, but the younger physicians wanted to wait and try persuasion. I wrote up the minutes of the meeting and gave them to the departmental secretary to type. Unfortunately, I had forgotten that she, too, was a Jehovah's Witness. She was, in fact, a minister of that sect. In no time at all, the family "went underground," as such families are known to do. They removed the child from the hospital and disappeared.

The next we heard about our little patient was that a neighbor had called the police, who took the child to Children's National Medical Center in the District of Columbia. The family was immediately taken to court, the child was treated appropriately, and the mother was placed under legal obligation to follow a regular schedule of clinic visits and to obtain treatment for him when needed. Interestingly, although we never saw the hemophilic child again, his mother later had another male child whom she brought to us to be tested for hemophilia. Fortunately, he turned out to be normal.

We were more successful in treating a ten-year-old boy whom we diagnosed with acute lymphoblastic leukemia. His single-parent mother refused treatment at Howard University Hospital, saying that she wanted to take him instead to a "faith healer." My chairman, Dr. Jenkins, agreed that we needed legal help. We called the District of Columbia Corporation Counsel and soon found ourselves in court. The boy, the mother, Dr. Jenkins, and I, each with a court appointed lawyer behind us, stood in a semi-circle before the judge. After hearing what each of us had to say, the judge pronounced his judgment that the boy should receive standard medical treatment. "The mother," he said, "can take herself to the faith healer!" We never saw the mother again. The child's grandfather brought him regularly to our outpatient clinic for care, and, fortunately, his leukemia went into remission and did not recur.

For both of the above children, the outcome was satisfactory, even though we had not managed the hemophilic child's situation very well.

There were two others whose parents refused treatment. A young black girl with histiocytosis was sent in by the juvenile court. Her disease was minimal and did not require specific treatment at the time. Although we insisted that the mother should continue to bring her in for regular visits, with the idea that the disease could worsen and treatment could be started immediately, mother and child disappeared and the patient was lost to follow up. The mother of an 18-month-old black boy diagnosed with neuroblastoma, a cancer that usually arises in the adrenal gland, wanted "diet therapy" for her son. The hospital had just hired a new legal counsel, and I was told to "stay out of it," that "he would take care of it." This child was also lost to follow up. We saw his death notice in the local newspaper a few months later. It was around that time that I became ready to retire. While these two cases were not the reason for my retirement, they helped me to decide that it was indeed time for me to go.

SPECIAL EFFORTS REQUIRED

In my ten years at Howard University, even though the total number of patients I saw was small, I encountered these four instances of refusal of therapy for serious diseases—diseases for which effective therapy was available. In my previous combined fifteen years, five in Oklahoma and almost ten in Michigan, I had encountered only one refusal. The lesson learned from this experience is that minority patients tend to be untrusting, and such situations require special efforts, not only from their pediatricians, but also from psychologists, social workers, legal counsel, and other team members who have expertise in working with minorities.

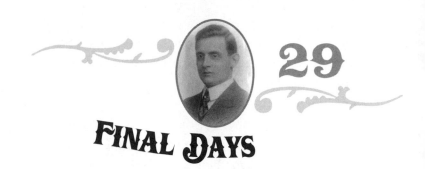

FINAL DAYS

*I*n 1940 many medical advances had yet to be discovered. Among the advances that awaited the future were antibiotics for the treatment of infections; vaccines for the prevention of poliomyelitis, measles, mumps, rubella, hemophilus, and hepatitis B; fluoridation of water for the prevention of dental caries; non-mercurial diuretics effective against high blood pressure and edema caused by heart failure; blood lipid-lowering agents; open heart surgery; cancer chemotherapy; knowledge of the immune system; and organ transplantation.

In the autumn of 1939, at 53 years of age, my father began to seem unsure of his actions and appeared to have an unusual pallor. As several months went by, this progressed to fumbling and an unsteady gait. Eventually he became unable to carry out his work with any degree of efficiency, and for a time his office nurse, Mary Goblirsch, performed many of the routine procedures and served as his driver when he made house calls.

DIAGNOSIS

By Christmas, it was clearly evident that "the doctor" was very ill, but no one seemed willing to mention it or do anything about it. My mother, a trained nurse, must have been so paralyzed with apprehension that she reacted with denial. The impasse was resolved when family friends Peter and Marie Cantine came to our house one evening and spoke to my father. "You have always taken care of us when we were sick," they said, "and now when you are sick we are going to take care of you." On December 20, the Cantines took my parents to the Mayo Clinic for my father's diagnostic studies, and after New Year's he returned to the Mayo Clinic so that an operation could be performed on his brain tumor.

CLINICAL COURSE

His Mayo Clinic record shows that he complained of visual difficulties, along with a right-sided headache. He had lost his ability to see anything on his left, the visual loss heralded by "blue flashes." He told the examining physician he thought his problems were caused by either a retinal hemorrhage or glaucoma—surely there was denial on his part. Loss of vision, restricting his ability to work, would have been extremely serious; but he must have been aware that his illness was much more devastating than that. Dr. W. McK. Craig, the neurosurgeon, performed a right craniotomy and decompression with partial removal of the right occipital lobe and a right temporo-occipital tumor. The tumor was a glioblastoma multiforme, the most malignant of brain tumors and the most common type found in adults. Because of its infiltrating nature, the tumor could not be completely excised. No radiotherapy was administered. After a rather slow convalescence, he was sent home from the hospital by ambulance on February 2, 1940.

The pressure on his brain caused by edema and the expanding tumor was temporarily relieved by the operation; his general condition improved for a while and then worsened as the tumor regrew. My mother switched into her nursing mode and cared for him at home, and during this time innumerable friends, neighbors, and former patients visited, brought food, and sent letters. The food included calves' brains sent especially for him by Mr. Fischer, the butcher, and a chocolate cake baked every week for all of us by the "Hotel Girls."

INFORMING THE CHILDREN

My mother was unable to talk to us children about how serious my father's illness was. After his first visit to Rochester, she told us, crying, that he had a tumor of the brain and that he would return to the Mayo Clinic for an operation. I remember saying to her, "Why, that's wonderful. They'll take out the tumor and he'll be all right!" Her response was to cry harder. After his surgery, he did improve for several months, and we children had every expectation that he would continue to get better. In retrospect, everyone in town but us knew that he would never get well, and I believe it was difficult for some of my school friends to refrain from telling me the truth. After those several months of improvement, his illness took a downhill course, but we children kept hoping that all would be well. My mother never talked to us about the eventual outcome. A few days before he died, Dr. Eaves, the physician who had assumed his practice, took the six of us aside and told us that he was dying.

HIS SHEEPSKIN

On one occasion my father sadly mentioned in my brother Paul's hearing that his "sheepskin" had been lost.

"Why no," said Paul. "It's hanging in the front closet, just as always!" Paul referred to the heavy sheepskin-lined coat that my father wore in the coldest winter weather.

"No, no," said my father. "I meant my medical school diploma. Once you lose your diploma, they never give you another one, you know."

The diploma had been stolen during his early years in practice, perhaps while he still had an office above the Goblirsch General Store. In fact, the family did obtain a copy of the diploma from the University of Minnesota at a much later date [Figure 13, on page 34].

FAMILY FINANCES

I overheard him, during his last illness, discussing his financial situation with a visitor. His bed had been moved to the living room downstairs so that his care would be easier and he would be more accessible to visitors. I had been kept home from school, in my final year of high school, because I had mumps, and they had obviously forgotten that I was upstairs. He wept and said to the visitor, "I have always been so concerned about the poor, and now my children will be the poorest of the poor!" The only other times I had ever heard him cry were at his parents' funerals.

He was referring to the Brey-Mahal grain elevator, which he was then building in Wabasso, in partnership with Joseph Mahal. Since Wabasso was located in the heart of a thriving agricultural area and he knew a good deal about grain, he had committed most of his money in this venture shortly before becoming ill. The village already had two grain elevators, and the Brey-Mahal elevator turned out to be a poor investment; in fact, it never became solvent. He had always carried a large life insurance coverage, believing that because he spent a great deal of time driving his automobile, he was at risk of death from a car accident. Unfortunately, most of the premiums were not paid during the long period when his health was failing. My mother, who was wholly absorbed in caring for him, had not found the time or energy to deal with finances, and somehow, neither the lawyers nor her relatives had helped her with this matter.

Our financial situation, while not by any means good, was not in fact as bad as he evidently thought. The house was paid for and in my mother's name. She paid off a residual mortgage on the farm with the small life insurance payments that came in. The tenant farmer, Frank Seikora, was both efficient and honest, and farm products were in demand as the Second World War was commencing. For the first time, the farm produced income—a big help with our college expenses. My mother went back to work as a psychiatric nurse. Both of my brothers spent time in the uniformed services, Al as a Navy pilot in training during the war, and Paul, who was too young to serve during the war, in the Army after the armistice. As military veterans, they received help with their college tuition. Tuition at the state university for the rest of us was not out of reach. Ann became a home economist, and I became a physician specializing in pediatric hematology and oncology. Virginia became a nurse, and Justine, a secretary. Al decided to become a farmer and settled on my father's farm outside Wabasso. Paul, after completing his university degree, worked first for the railroad company and later in retail sales.

BURIAL

For my father's funeral, St. Anne's Catholic Church overflowed with people who had come to pay their respects, and a public address system had to be installed for those who could not find seating in the church. The public address system was installed by Francis W. Hirsch, the first baby my father had delivered when he first came to Wabasso. Mr. Hirsch was named for him, and my dad always took a special interest in young Francis W. Dr. Brey was buried in the Catholic cemetery south of Wabasso.

WABASSO PUBLIC SCHOOL YEAR BOOK OBITUARY

My father, who greatly enjoyed helping children and cared passionately about promoting education, would have been pleased that the 1940 Wabasso Public School yearbook, *The White Rabbit*, was dedicated to him. Wallace F. Simpson, the school principal, wrote in it the following tribute:

"This volume is dedicated to the memory of a man who labored patiently to build a strong educational program for his community. His untimely death cut short a life of service to his fellow men.

"Words are inadequate instruments to convey expressions of thought reflecting the memory picture of a friend departed. The late Dr. F. W. Brey, M. D., was a friend. He was a true friend. The services that he rendered no man can measure. Of him it can truly be said that he added to the measure of happiness and relieved suffering and made life's pathway brighter by the work he did.

"Dr. F. W. Brey, M. D., was a member of the Wabasso School Board from 1929 to 1940. He was president of the school board from 1932 to 1940.

"Dr. Brey was born March 22, 1886, and died June 8, 1940."

OTHER OBITUARIES

Two news clippings, evidently from the *Wabasso Standard*, that were found in Aunt Anne's scrapbook after her death, are included as Appendix F.

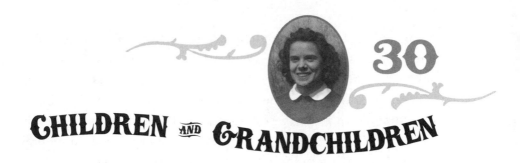

CHILDREN AND GRANDCHILDREN

ow, at 82 years of age, I look back over a long life that includes almost 60 years of marriage to Fran [Figure 66], living in five states (Minnesota, Illinois, Oklahoma, Michigan, and Maryland), and more than 50 years of practicing medicine. I can say that I believe my most important contribution, certainly the accomplishment which gives me greatest satisfaction, is that Fran and I have three wonderful children and seven bright and happy grandchildren, as well as a lovely daughter-in-law and two stalwart sons-in-law.

We returned to our roots in retirement, and we live in Rochester, Minnesota, in a continuing care retirement community managed by the Mayo Clinic and located just one block from the Mayo Clinic. Here we enjoy, among other amenities, the opportunity to attend many of the Mayo medical/scientific teaching sessions. We still do a little work and a bit of writing in our respective fields. It is our greatest pleasure that Carol, along with Stuart and their two daughters, lives in Plymouth, a suburb of Minneapolis and visits us often. Four of my siblings live in Minnesota, the fifth one lives in Wisconsin, and other relatives are not too far away. Most of Fran's relatives left Minnesota long ago and are now situated in California, Nevada, and Arizona.

Rick [Figure 67] is a professor of family practice at the University of Louisville in Louisville, Kentucky. His wife, Cheryl, is a nurse and homemaker. Carol [Figure 68] is a nurse in a Minneapolis day surgery clinic and an artist. Her husband, Stuart, is an electrical engineer. Alice [Figure 69] is an associate professor of physical chemistry at the University of North Carolina in Greensboro, and her husband, Ed, is an assistant professor of physics at the same university. Rick and Cheryl have four children, Kari, a fourth-year student at the University of Illinois; Jennifer, in her second year at St. Olaf College; Michael, a junior in high school; and Sarah, a seventh grader. Carol and Stuart have two daughters, Jessie, who finished her first year at St. Cloud State University, and Rachel, who is a junior in high school. Alice and Ed's daughter, Deborah, is in the sixth grade. We look forward to seeing what all of them will be doing in the future.

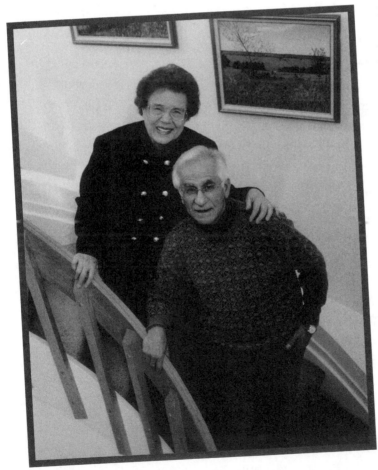

Fig. 66: *Fran and Terry Haddy at home in Potomac, Maryland, 2001.*

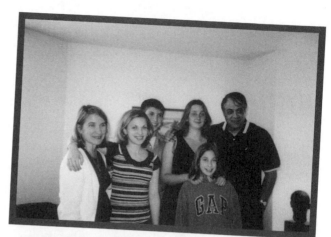

Fig. 67: *Rick and Cheryl Haddy with their children (from left to right, Cheryl, Jenni, Michael, Kari, and Rick, with Sarah in front), 2003.*

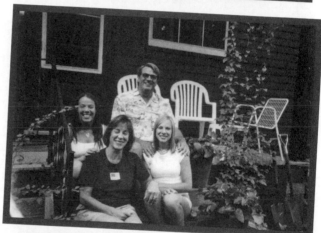

Fig. 68: *Carol and Stuart Froelich with Jessica (left) and Rachel (right), 2005.*

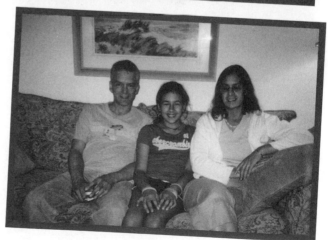

Fig. 69: *Alice and Ed Hellen with Deborah (center), 2005.*

GLOSSARY

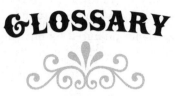

ACETAMINOPHEN. Tylenol. A non-prescription drug that relieves pain and fever, similar to aspirin, but with weaker anti-inflammatory effects.

ACETYLSALICYLIC ACID. Aspirin.

ANESTHESIA. Loss of the ability to feel pain, caused by a drug or other medical intervention.

ANGINA PECTORIS. Chest pain, often radiating to the arms, especially the left arm, usually caused by inadequate oxygen being supplied to the heart muscle.

ANTIBIOTIC. A chemical substance produced by microorganisms that inhibits or kills other microorganisms, used to treat infections and also cancers.

ANTIGEN. A substance that is capable of inducing a specific immune response.

ANTIRACHITIC. Effective in the prevention of rickets.

ANTISEPSIS. Any procedure that reduces the numbers of microbes and inhibits their growth and development but does not necessarily kill them.

ANTITOXIN. An antibody against a toxin. Specific antitoxins against bacteria are obtained from immunized animals and are usually used for prevention, less commonly for treatment of infection.

APPENDECTOMY. Surgical removal of the appendix.

APPENDICITIS. Inflammation of the appendix.

ASEPSIS. Any procedure that prevents contact with microbes.

ASPIRIN. Acetylsalicylic acid. A drug that relieves pain and fever and has anti-inflammatory effects.

BACTERIA. Single-cell microorganisms, rod-shaped or spherical, that can cause disease.

CADAVER. A dead body, often one that is preserved for dissection.

CARBOLIC ACID. Phenol. An antiseptic.

CATHARTIC. Also, purgative. An agent that causes evacuation of the bowels.

CHILDBED FEVER. Puerperal fever. A specific contagious infection passed by direct contact, usually by the physician, to maternity patients. Fatal septicemia frequently resulted. Oliver Wendell Holmes first proposed that this disease was contagious, and his theory was confirmed by Ignaz Philipp Semmelweis.

COMMUNICABLE DISEASE. Infectious disease. Disease that is capable of being transmitted.

CONGESTIVE HEART FAILURE. A clinical syndrome caused by heart disease, with symptoms of shortness of breath and/or edema due to congestion in the lungs and/or peripheral blood circulation.

COWPOX VACCINE. A mild, self-limited skin disease of milk cows caused by cowpox virus. The English physician Edward Jenner first demonstrated in 1798 that inoculation with material from cowpox lesions conferred immunity against smallpox.

CUPPING. Application to the skin of a small glass cup from which air had been evacuated by heating, for the purpose of drawing blood to the surface of the body in order to cause irritation or for bloodletting.

CYANOSIS. A bluish color, especially of the skin and mucous membranes.

CYSTOSCOPIC EXAMINATION. Direct visual examination of the bladder with a cystoscope.

DIURETIC. An agent that increases the excretion of urine.

EDEMA. The accumulation of excessive amounts of fluid in the tissues of the body. Most commonly beneath the skin, but other tissues such as the lung can also be affected.

EMETIC. Agent that causes vomiting.

ENCEPHALITIS. Inflammation of the brain.

ENDEMIC. A disease or agent present or usually prevalent at all times in a population or geographical area.

EPIDEMIC. An outbreak of disease that affects many people in a community or region at one time. Usually refers to infection but could also refer to any other health-related event.

ETIOLOGY. The cause or origin of a disease or disorder.

GASTROENTERITIS. Inflammation of the stomach and intestines. Can cause loss of appetite, nausea, vomiting, diarrhea, and/or abdominal pain.

GERM THEORY. Also, the animalculae theory. Cotton Mather postulated that specific microorganisms passed from one individual to another by towels or direct contact could invade the body, multiply inside the tissues, and cause certain diseases. He recognized that such invasions did not always cause disease.

GOITER. Enlargement of the thyroid gland, with resultant visible swelling of the front of the neck.

GRIPPE. Also, *la grippe*. Influenza. The term is rarely used in modern times.

HEMANGIOMA. A benign tumor made up of blood vessels.

HEPARIN. An anticoaglulant, used to prevent blood clotting.

HERNIA. The protrusion of a loop of an organ or tissue through an abnormal opening. An inguinal hernia is a loop of intestine that leaves the abdomen through the inguinal ring and forms a bulge in the groin.

HEROIC THERAPY. The heroic school of therapy, which flourished before the twentieth century, advocated vigorous bleeding, blistering, purging, vomiting, and sweating, often to the patient's detriment.

HOOKWORM. A parasitic roundworm that enters through the skin and infects the gastro-intestinal tract.

HYPOXIA. Reduced oxygen supply to tissues of the body.

HYSTERECTOMY. Surgical removal of the uterus.

IDIOPATHIC. Of unknown cause.

IMMUNIZE. Also, immunization. To protect against infectious disease.

INFECTIOUS DISEASE. Communicable disease. Disease that is capable of being transmitted.

ISLETS OF LANGERHANS. Microscopic structures in the pancreas that are responsible for the endocrine function of producing insulin and other hormones.

INTOXICANTS. Usually alcohol. Cause impaired mental or physical functioning.

KYPHOSIS. Also, humpback or hunchback. Convex curvature of the spine as viewed from the side.

LIGATE. To tie or bind with a ligature.

LIGATURE. Material, such as cotton, silk, catgut, or wire, used to tie a blood vessel or a segment of tissue.

MCBURNEY'S POINT. A point half-way between the right iliac crest and the umbilicus. Tenderness at this point is an indication that the appendix is inflamed.

MICROBES, MICROORGANISMS. Organisms of extremely small size, visualized only with the aid of a microscope. Included in this category are bacteria, viruses, fungi, and protozoa.

MYOCARDITIS. Inflammation of the heart muscle.

MYRINGOTOMY. An incision in the ear drum.

NARCOTICS. Usually opiates such as morphine. Cause insensibility or stupor.

NEUROLOGICAL. Also, neurologic. Pertaining to nerves.

NEUROSIS. Disorder in which the symptoms are distressing but reality is intact, behavior does not violate social norms, and there is no apparent organic cause.

OOPHORECTOMY. Surgical removal of an ovary or ovaries.

PANDEMIC. An epidemic becomes a pandemic when many cases occur throughout the world within a short time.

PARASITE. An organism which lives upon or within another living organism, at some advantage to itself.

PATENT DUCTUS ARTERIOSUS. A blood vessel connecting the left pulmonary artery to the descending aorta in the fetus, which fails to close at birth.

PELLAGRA. A condition caused by deficiency of niacin, one of the B vitamins.

PENICILLIN. Natural or synthetic antibiotics derived from the fungus *Penicillium*, which kill a variety of bacteria.

PNEUMONIA. Inflammation of the lungs. Also, bronchopneumonia, inflammation of the bronchi.

PSYCHOSIS. A mental disorder characterized by gross impairment of reality or inability to meet the ordinary demands of life.

PURGATIVE. Also, cathartic. An agent that causes evacuation of the bowels.

PURGE. To cause evacuation of the bowels.

RALES. Also, crackles. Abnormal, discontinuous, nonmusical sounds heard upon auscultation of the chest.

RESPIRATORY. Refers to the function of breathing.

RESURRECTIONIST. Also, body snatcher or "sack-em-up-man." Professional grave robbers who sold bodies to medical schools for a fee.

RHINITIS. Inflammation of the mucous membrane of the nose, usually with a discharge.

RICKETS. A disorder of bony development caused by a variety of vitamin D, calcium, and phosphorus deficiencies.

SCURVY. A condition caused by deficiency of ascorbic acid, vitamin C, and characterized by weakness, anemia, spongy gums, a tendency to bleed, and induration of the leg muscles.

SEPTICEMIA. Also, blood poisoning. Systemic disease associated with the presence of pathogenic microorganisms or their toxins in the blood.

SHOCK. Profound failure of the circulation to maintain blood flow through the vital organs.

SPONTANEOUS GENERATION. The theory that diseases could be spontaneously originated, or that diseases could arise *de novo*, without the transmission of specific material from pre-existing cases.

STERILITY. Freedom from microbes accomplished by physical methods (heat), chemicals (formaldehyde, alcohol), radiation, or mechanical methods (filtration).

SUBCLINICAL. Without symptoms or signs of a disease, often the early stages or the very mild form of a disease.

SULFA DRUGS. Also, sulfonamides. Derivatives of sulfanilamide, which inhibit folic acid synthesis in microorganisms and kill bacteria.

TAPEWORM. A parasitic, segmented flatworm that attaches to the wall of the intestine.

TOXEMIA OF PREGNANCY. Eclampsia. Convulsions occurring in a pregnant woman before, or within two or three weeks after, delivery of an infant. Associated with preecampsia, which is characterized by high blood pressure, the presence of protein in the urine, and edema.

TOXIC SHOCK SYNDROME. A severe illness caused by infection and characterized by high fever of sudden onset, hypotension, and shock. Vomiting, diarrhea, myalgia (muscle pain), and a sunburn-like rash with peeling of the skin, especially the palms and soles, may be present.

TOXINS. Also, toxic chemicals. Poisons.

TOXOID. A modified bacterial toxin that is not toxic but can combine with an antitoxin or stimulate the formation of an antitoxin.

TRICHINOSIS. Infestation with trichinella, a parasitic round worm found coiled in the muscles of pigs and other infected animals, which infects humans when meat is improperly cooked.

TYLENOL. Acetaminophen.

VACCINE. A suspension of weakened or killed microorganisms administered for the prevention or treatment of disease.

VARICOSE VEINS. Enlarged and tortuous veins, usually involving the veins of the lower extremities but can be anywhere in the body.

VIRUSES. Microorganisms too small to be seen with an ordinary microcope, can cause disease.

VITAMIN. A general term for a number of unrelated substances that are present in foods and are needed in small amounts for normal functioning of the body.

APPENDICES

APPENDIX A.

THE DEPARTMENT OF MEDICINE, UNIVERSITY OF MINNESOTA.

The first (unpaid) medical faculty members at the University of Minnesota were physicians who were in private practice. They were appointed to the College of Medicine, and they performed an examining, not a teaching, service. They functioned as the state board of medical examiners from 1883 to 1887, and as such they were responsible for issuing certificates to practice medicine to graduates of approved medical schools and to persons who passed an examination given by the board. Physicians who had been in practice for more than five years previous to 1883 were exempt from the requirements for licensure. Members of the board could refuse to grant or revoke licenses for unprofessional or dishonorable conduct. They also conducted the entrance examination for the medical school.

MERGER OF THE MEDICAL SCHOOLS

The university medical school was organized as a teaching body in 1888 when two previously existing schools joined the university's Department of Medicine. The Minnesota Hospital College in Minneapolis and the St. Paul Medical College in St. Paul merged with the College of Medicine to form the College of Medicine and Surgery, and their students became students at the new university school. The Minnesota Hospital College offered its building at Sixth Street and Ninth Avenue South for the temporary use of the students, and the offer was accepted. The third previously existing school, the Minneapolis College of Physicians and Surgeons (Hamline University's medical department) remained outside the group for a time but became part of the University of Minnesota in 1908. After this final merger was accomplished, there was only one medical school in Minnesota until many years later, when the Mayo Medical School was established in Rochester, Minnesota.

THE COLLEGE OF MEDICINE AND SURGERY

The College of Medicine and Surgery was to have nine departments with a professor for each department and the president of the university serving as the tenth faculty member. The departments included anatomy and physiology, pathology, materia medica and therapeutics, medical chemistry, preventive medicine (personal and public hygiene), practice of medicine, surgery, obstetrics and diseases of women and children, and diseases of the nervous system and medical jurisprudence. The university decided that faculty members who taught the basic sciences of chemistry, anatomy, physiology, and pathology, as well as the dean, who was also a professor of surgery, should be paid salaries by the university. All other teachers were unpaid volunteers, the usual practice in the medical schools of the time. The College of Medicine and Surgery started out as a three year training school but soon became a four year school, and before long an additional academic requirement of first one year and then two years of undergraduate education was added.

For its first few years, the medical school had occupied the building of the Minnesota Hospital College located at Sixth Street and Ninth Avenue South in Minneapolis. The first building on campus was dedicated as Medical Hall in 1892. Re-named Millard Hall in 1906, Medical Hall later became the Pharmacy Building and still later, Wulling Hall. The Medical Chemistry Building (known as the "Bowling Alley" because of its length) was completed in 1892 or 1893. The one-story east end of the building, which accounted for its nickname, contained student laboratories for histology, embryology, and bacteriology, and here the students learned how to examine materials for these areas of interest and how to prepare tissue slides, culture bacteria, and stain bacteria. When the Laboratory of Medical Sciences (later re-named Wesbrook Hall) was completed in 1895, it housed histology, pathology, bacteriology, and physiology. The Anatomy Building was constructed in 1900 but was unfortunately gutted by fire in 1902 and destroyed by fire in 1908 or 1910. The Institute of Public Health and Pathology, completed in 1907, contained both the university's Department of Pathology and the laboratory of the State Board of Health.

Students initially gained outpatient experience in a free dispensary located on the university campus. This was replaced in 1900 by the College of Medicine and Surgery Dispensary at 1908 Washington Avenue, on the west bank of the Mississippi River at Seven Corners. The university controlled the St. Paul Free Dispensary, and held clinics as well in almost all the hospitals in Minneapolis and St. Paul. Although Elliott Memorial Hospital did not open until 1911, the university hospital actually began in 1909 with patients being admitted to beds in a group of houses located at 200 and 304 State Street and at 300 and 304 Washington Avenue in southeast Minneapolis. The large house at 303 Washington Avenue was equipped to take care of 34 surgical and obstetrical patients and was the first university hospital.

APPENDIX B.

Biographical Sketch of Dr. Frank W. Brey, by Henry A. Castle, who wrote, in his *History of Minnesota*, published in 1915, the following:

> *The leading physician in point of patronage and recognized ability at Wabasso is Dr. Frank W. Brey, who has his degree as Doctor of Medicine from the University of Minnesota and has been identified with this section of the state as a physician and surgeon for the past five years.*
>
> *Dr. Frank W. Brey was born in Lafayette Township, Nicollet County, Minnesota, March 23, 1886. His father is Alois Brey, who was born in Austria [both of my paternal grandparents were born in Neumarkt, Germany. Because Germany was then part of the Austro-Hungarian Empire, they listed themselves in the United States census as being born in Austria] in 1854, emigrated to the United States in 1873, locating in Nicollet County, and was an independent farmer there from 1881 until he retired, his home now being in New Ulm. Alois Brey married Anna Altmann, also a native of Austria. They are the parents of a family of six children, as follows: Alois, who conducts a cafe in Springfield, Minnesota [later, when I knew him, Uncle Louie was the owner and operator of a farm in Nicollet County]; Anton, living on the old homestead farm in Nicollet County; Joseph, who is a veterinary surgeon at Stella, Nebraska; Dr. Frank W.; Theresa, wife of Anton Goblirsch, a farmer in Nicollet County; and Mary, wife of Andrew Kleisner [Gleisner], on a farm in Nicollet County.*
>
> *Dr. Frank W. Brey received a common school education in Sibley County, was graduated from the New Ulm High School with the class of 1905 and soon afterwards entered the medical department of the University of Minnesota, receiving his degree of M. D. after completing the course with the class of 1910. While in the university Doctor Brey became affiliated with the medical fraternity of the Alpha Kappa Kappa.*

Wabasso was the point selected for the beginning of his practice and since 1910 he has been steadily progressing in reputation and experience and now enjoys a large general practice both in medicine and surgery.

Doctor Brey is a member of the County and Minnesota State Medical societies and the American Medical Association. In April, 1913, he was appointed county coroner, and on November 3, 1914, was regularly elected to that office for a period of four years. Politically he is a democrat and is a member of the Catholic Church. Doctor Brey has some business interests outside of his profession, including the holding of some stock in the Twin City Fire Insurance Company. He is unmarried.

APPENDIX G.

A chronological list of Redwood County certificates of death signed by Dr. F. W. Brey and found among his papers.

Date of Death Township/Town	Name	Age/Sex	Occupation	Cause of Death
May 23, 1914 Lamberton	GG	20M	Farmer	Strangulation/hanging Suicide
June 23, 1914 Sherman	SN	50M	Laborer	Compound fracture of skull Accident/wagon wheels
July 14, 1914	ME	3 mo F	None	Marasmus/asthenia
July 17, 1914	FO	6F	None	Compound fracture of skull Accident/manure Spreader
Nov 6, 1915 North Hero	HP	23M	Farmer	Shotgun wound skull Suicide
Dec 23, 1915 Sheridan	LF	11M	—	Bullet wound of brain Accident
Jan 10, 1916 Sheridan	EH	83F	None	Arteriosclerosis
Jan 11, 1916	RB	—	—	Shotgun to abdomen Inquest unnecessary

Date of Death Township/Town	Name	Age/Sex	Occupation	Cause of Death
Feb 7, 1916 Lucan	JF	58M	—	Cerebral hemorrhage
Jun 16, 1916 Sanborn	ES	2 moM	None	Bronchopneumonia
Nov 13, 1916 Swedes Forest	RT	58F	Housework	Influenza
Dec 22, 1916 Vesta	W	78F	Housework	Cerebral hemorrhage Inquest unnecessary
Dec 24, 1916 Seaforth	OG	54M	Railroad brakeman	Fracture of neck, crushing of chest, fell from moving freight car
Nov 1, 1917 West —	WB	28-	—	Fracture base of skull Automobile accident
Mar 13, 1919 Redwood Falls	GL	47M	Farmer	Strangulation/hanging Suicide
July 31, 1919 Sheridan	FH	79M	Farmer	Strangulation/hanging Suicide
Dec 4, 1919 Springdale	WR	19M	Farm labor	Shotgun wound neck Accident
Apr 29, 1920 Charlestown	JB	—	—	Crushed skull and cranium RR collision
Apr 29, 1920 Charlestown	C	—	Train conductor	—
May 22, 1920 Willow Lake	JR	79M	Farmer	—
Apr 25, 1921 Sherman	HK	87M	Retired laborer	Strangulation/hanging
Feb 11, 1922 Sherman	OF	—	—	Born dead
Oct 28, 1922 Sherman	MS	63F	Common housework	Cerebral hemorrhage

APPENDIX D.

Medical Abstracts* and reprints found among Dr. Frank W. Brey's papers.

HEMORRHOIDS

1. Anderson, H. G., and others. Discussion on the treatment of hemorrhoids by injection. *Proceedings of the Royal Society of Medicine*, Section of Surgery 17:75-77, February, 1924.

2. Calvo, T. Treatment of hemorrhoids by interstitial injections of urea and double bichlorhydrate of quinin [sic]. *Revista de Medicina of Cirugia* 30:1192-1197, March, 1925 (No. 39044).

3. Watson, Leigh F. The office treatment of hemorrhoids. *Chicago Medical Recorder* 47:93-96, March, 1926 (No. 37622).

4. Mantague, J. F. How to make a snapshot diagnosis of hemorrhoids. *Medical Journal and Record* 121:770, June, 1925 (No. 38810).

5. Crowe, Harold E. The injection treatment for hemorrhoids. *The China Medical Journal* 40:417-419, May, 1926 (No. 45419).

6. Deavor, T. L. The two clamp method of removing hemorrhoids: a new and simple procedure. *American Journal of Surgery* 50:193-197, October, 1926 (No. 51247).

7. Campbell, Frederick B. Injection treatment for hemorrhoids. *The Journal of the Kansas Medical Society* 27:9-10, January, 1927 (No. 60746).

8. Deutsch, William F. Electro-coagulation of hemorrhoids. *The American Journal of Physical Therapy* 3:500-501, February, 1927 (No. 61079).

9. Rolfe, William A. The treatment of internal hemorrhoids with quinine and urea hydrochloride. *The New England Journal of Medicine* 198:187-188, March, 1928 (No. 6584).

10. Buie, L. A. Injection treatment of hemorrhoids. *Proceedings of Staff Meetings of the Mayo Clinic* 5:43-44, February 1930.

   * Articles followed by numbers were included in two books of abstracts.

VARICOSE VEINS

1. Stebbing, George F. Modern technique in treatment: treatment of varicose ulcers. *The Lancet* 212:886-887, April, 1927 (No. 70828).

2. McPheeters, H. O. The injection treatment of varicose veins by the use of sclerosing solutions. *Surgery, Gynecology and Obstetrics* 45:541-547, October, 1927 (No. 68100).

3. McKim, L. H. The present status of the treatment of varicose veins by injection. *The Canadian Medical Association Journal* 19:578-580, November, 1928 (No. 73426).

4. Thornhill, Ronald. The treatment of varicose veins by injection methods. *The Practitioner* 120:54-58, January, 1928 (No. 62761).

5. Crivelli, L. Results of injection treatment of varicose veins. *The Medical Journal of Australia* 1:139, February, 1929 (No. 490).

6. Hanschell, H. M. Notes on the injection treatment of varicose veins. *The British Medical Journal* 3508:542-543, March, 1928 (No. 67089).

7. Marcovici, Eugene E. An efficient treatment for varicose ulcers. *Archives of Dermatology and Syphilology* 18:290, August, 1928 (No. 70434).

8. Bratrud, Arthur F. The injection treatment of varicose veins. *Minnesota Medicine*, pp. 33-39, January, 1929.

9. Dixon, C. F., and Counseller, V. S. The results of the injection treatment of varicose veins. *Proceedings of the Staff Meetings of the Mayo Clinic* 5:42-43, February, 1930.

10. Logefeil, Rudolph C. Varicose veins: some special considerations in treatment. *Minnesota Medicine* 15:172-180, March, 1932.

    * Articles followed by numbers were included in two books of abstracts.

APPENDIX E.

Partial list* of medical textbooks in Dr. Frank W. Brey's library.

INTERNAL MEDICINE

1. Forchheimer, Frederick. *The Prophylaxis and Treatment of Internal Disease: Designed for the Use of Practitioners and of Advanced Students of Medicine*, 2nd ed. D. Appleton & Co., New York, 1910.

2. Forchheimer, Frederick. *Therapeusis of Internal Diseases*, vols. I-V. D. Appleton & Co., New York, 1913.

3. Osler, Sir William. *The Principles and Practice of Medicine: Designed for the Use of Practitioners and Students of Medicine*, 8th ed. D. Appleton & Co., New York, 1914.

4. Sahli, Prof. Dr. Hermann. *A Treatise on Diagnostic Methods of Examination*, 2nd ed. W. B. Saunders Co., Philadelphia, 1914.

5. Einhorn, Max. *Diseases of the Stomach: A Text-Book for Practitioners and Students*, 6th ed. William Wood & Co., New York, 1917.

NEUROPSYCHIATRY

6. Church, Archibald, and Peterson, Frederick. *Nervous and Mental Diseases*, 6th ed. W. B. Saunders Co., Philadelphia, 1910.

DERMATOLOGY

7. Stellwagon, Henry W. *Treatise on Diseases of the Skin; for the Use of Advanced Students and Practitioners*, 6th ed. W. B. Saunders Co., Philadelphia, 1910.

ORTHOPEDICS

8. Scudder, Charles Locke. *The Treatment of Fractures: with Notes upon a Few Common Dislocations*, 6th ed. W. B. Saunders Co., Philadelphia, 1910.

9. Sluss, John W. *Emergency Surgery: for the General Practitioner*, 2nd ed. P. Blakiston's Son & Co., Philadelphia, 1911.

10. Keen, William Williams. *Surgery: Its Principles and Practice by Various Authors*, vol III. W. B. Saunders Co., Philadelphia, 1914.

11. McPheeters, H. O. *Varicose Veins: with Special Reference to the Injection Treatment*, 2nd ed. F. A. Davis Co., Philadelphia, 1930.

12. Ballenger, William Lincoln. *Diseases of the Nose, Throat, and Ear: Medical and Surgical*, 4th ed., Lea & Febeiger, Philadelphia, 1914.

OBSTETRICS

13. Hirst, Barton Cooke. *A Text-Book of Obstetrics*, 8th ed. W. B. Saunders Co., Philadelphia, 1918.

PEDIATRICS

14. Chapin, Henry Dwight, and Pisek, Godfrey Roger. *Diseases of Infants and Children*, 2nd ed. William Wood & Co., New York, 1911.

15. Kerley, Charles Gilmore. *The Practice of Pediatrics*. W. B. Saunders Co., Philadelphia, 1915.

16. Hess, Julius H. *Feeding and Nutritional Disorders of Infancy and Childhood*, 4th ed. F. A. Davis & Co., Philadelphia, 1925.

17. Holt, L. Emmett, and Howland, John. *The Diseases of Infancy and Childhood: for the Use of Students and Practitioners of Medicine*, 7th ed. D. Appleton & Co., New York, 1917.

*A number of his newer and more valuable books were sold along with the practice after his death in 1940.

APPENDIX F.

Obituaries. Two news clippings, evidently from the *Wabasso Standard*, found in Aunt Anne M. Daub's scrapbook after her death, are reproduced here.

DEATH OF DR. F. W. BREY CLOSES ACTIVE CAREER;

SERVICES HELD TUESDAY

Resolution

The following resolution was adopted by the Board of Education of Wabasso public school district 84, Wabasso, Minnesota.

With deep sorrow the Board of Education of Wabasso public school district 84 records the death, on Saturday, June 8th, 1940, of Dr. F. W. Brey, since 1929 a member and chairman of the Board, and extends heartfelt sympathy to Mrs. Brey and other members of the family. For many years Dr. Brey has been actively interested in the welfare of this community, especially as affecting the family. This experience, added to the sense of human needs and values, particularly fitted him for the presidency of the School Board, and his service in that office was marked by clear insight, keen wisdom, and loyalty to Wabasso's educational needs.

He contributed to the present high standards of education in our community and his death deprives this Board of a courageous and trusted leader, and Wabasso of a worthy citizen whose work for those who are distressed and afflicted will stand as a lasting memorial.

L.A. Torney, vice president

C. H. Leistikow, clerk

Elmer E. Franta, treasurer

L. A. Bangerter, director

Carl Radel, director

(Editor's note—The above resolution was tendered Mrs. Elizabeth Brey by the Board)

PROMINENT CITIZEN WAS PHYSICIAN HERE 30 YEARS SUCCUMBED TO BRAIN TUMOR EARLY SATURDAY MORNING; HUNDREDS PAY RESPECTS

The greatest Physician of all healed for all time the lingering illness of Dr F. W. Brey, M. D., when he was relieved of his earthly ailments at 4:30 a.m. Saturday, June 8. Death came after a protracted illness of nearly nine months. The doctor suffered from a brain tumor from which all of modern medical science could offer no recovery.

Funeral services were conducted for his remains Tuesday morning at 9 a.m. from the church of which he had been a member for the 30 years he had practiced his profession in Wabasso, St. Annes's Catholic Church, with Rev. P. F. Remskar in charge. Burial was in St. Anne's cemetery here. In tribute to his memory, floral offerings were profuse and many persons were denied admittance to the church edifice due to insufficient room, attesting [to] the high esteem in which he was held by his fellow citizens and those from other communities. During the hour of the service, from 8:30 to 10 a.m., business places closed in respect to a departed fellow business man.

Rev. William Neudecker of Stewart, a friend of the family, was present in the sanctuary.

CITIZEN, DOCTOR

As a young man, fresh from his alma mater, Dr. Frank Brey came to this community filled with a deep sense of duty toward mankind and this ideal he kept always before him. It is no small task to write about a man who stood out as he did among his fellow men.

Those early times were trying days. Deep snow often caused him to walk long distances to farm homes; where horses failed to pass through the drifted roads he pushed through to aid some suffering soul. He learned the value of tenacity and gifted with a strong heart, stuck to his job. It has been said by those that knew him that in the nearly 30 years he practiced here, not once until just recent years did he leave his office to take any vacation for himself.

With the founding of his home and the coming responsibility of rearing a family, he devoted himself unselfishly to his children and found in them what relaxation he was accorded.

For the years he was associated with other members on the school board of district 84, he served as a leader; known to be progressive, he believed solidly in good education for the children and young people of this community. Likewise, he was a firm believer in home institutions.

The doctor had diagnosed his own case. He realized he was suffering from an illness from which he might not recover. He first went to Rochester, Minn., on December 18, 1939, where he submitted to an examination. After remaining there two weeks he returned home. He picked his pallbearers from among his friends. He returned again to Rochester on January 17 and submitted to an operation January 22 for the relief of his malady but medical aid was unavailing. After several days he returned home. During all that time he was never left alone. Someone was with him constantly, and especially so during the last week of his illness when his life began to ebb slowly and it was only a matter of hours until he would be Crossing the Bar.

Those who were close to him knew that he worked hard and conscientiously, perhaps too much so and as the clergy stated at his last rites, many were able to attend only because of the attention he had given them at some bygone time. He was the only doctor who remained at his post in this village until he was physically unable to do so.

WABASSO STANDARD OBITUARY

Frank W. Brey was born in Lafayette township, Nicollet county, near New Ulm, on March 22, 1886. He was reared in that community and as a youth attended and was graduated from the New Ulm high school in 1904. He was the son of Alois and Anna Brey.

Following his high school graduation, he attended the University of Minnesota, where he chose to study for the medical profession. Upon completion of his course in 1910, he came to Wabasso, then a small village only ten years old, and set up his medical practice. Having thus spent the last 30 years in this, his home community, he saw it grow and prosper and took an active part in civic life.

On November 24, 1921, he was united in marriage with Elizabeth K. Daub at St. Anne's church. To this union was born six children, all of whom with their mother, survive him. The children are Anna Catherine, 17, Theresa E., 16, Alois, 15, Virginia, 13, Paul, 12, and Justine, 11.

Beside his immediate family, he is survived by two sisters and three brothers, namely, Mrs. Anton (Theresa) Goblirsch, Lafayette; Mrs. Andrew (Mary) Gleisner, Fairfax; Alois, New Ulm; Anton, Lafayette; and Dr. J. H. Brey, Nebraska City, Nebr. Also mourning his death are many other friends and relatives.

During his career, he had served as a member of the Wabasso school board for the past 12 years in the capacity of president of the body. For practically the time of his residence here he had served as health officer for the village. Widening his scope, he served three terms as Redwood county coroner from 1915 to the end of his term in 1926.

He had affiliated with St. George Catholic Aid Society, the Catholic Order of Foresters, was a member of the American Medical Association, had been elected to the Alpha Kappa Kappa fraternity at the University of Minnesota and carried memberships in the Wabasso Commercial Club and the local chapter of the Izaak Walton League of America. For several years past, up to the time of his illness, he was a partner in the firm of the Brey-Mahal elevator.

It had been his wish before his death that the following serve as his pall-bears: Fred Fixsen, Seaforth; George Fixsen, Peter Cantine, Wabasso; Charles Gores, Wanda; John Bradish, Marshall; and George Neudecker, Clements.

With a feeling that his loss was not only his family's but the community's as well, there can be no regret for the manifestation of his Maker's Will. A useful life has come to its ultimate close and those who mourn about his former family altar have the knowledge of the community's deep sympathy in their present sorrow.

Those from a distance who attended the funeral were Father Neudecker, Stewart; Mr. and Mrs. Anton Brey, Jr., Mr. and Mrs. Anton Brey, Sr., Mr. and Mrs. Norbert Brey, Mr. and Mrs. Anton Goblirsch and daughter Stella, son Paul, Mrs. Helen Brey, Mr. and Mrs. Ed Altmann, Dr. and Mrs. H. J. Just, Mr. and Mrs. Jos. G. Meidl of Lafayette; Mr. and Mrs. Alfred Aschenbrenner and family, Mr. and Mrs. Albert Bauer and daughter DeLoris, Mr. and Mrs. Frank Altmann, Mrs. Geo. Pechtel, Mr. and Mrs. John Altmann, Mrs. Charles Altmann, Mrs. Barbara Stadick, Mrs. Emil Hacker, Mr. and Mrs. Frank J. Byer, Mr. and Mrs. Leslie Schreyer, Alois P. Brey, Mrs. Ted Miller, Mr. and Mrs. Al Martinka, Mrs. Jos. Martinka, Mr. and Mrs. Max Byli of New Ulm; Mr. and Mrs. M. B. Fenno and family of Danube; Mr. and Mrs. Jos. Brey of Winona; Mrs. Paul Zeug and Neil of Elmwood, Wis.; Mrs. Thomas Taylor of St. Joseph, Mich.; Mr. and Mrs. Robert Hughes and daughter Norma, Mrs. Cora Meyers of Mankato; Dr. A. P. Goblirsch of Sleepy Eye; Dr. and Mrs. Grey, Mr. and Mrs. John Bradish and daughter Elaine, Mrs. Arthur Amann of Marshall; Dr. and Mrs. J. H. Brey of Nebraska City, Nebr.; and Mr. and Mrs. Henry Goblirsch and family of Gary, So. Dak.

There were many others from the above and other nearby towns whose names it was impossible to obtain.